HIV in South Africa

T0252591

Of approximately 39.5 million HIV positive people in the world, 24.7 million live in sub-Saharan Africa, and 5.5 million South Africans are HIV positive. South Africa, despite its relatively powerful economy and infrastructure, has been dramatically affected by the HIV pandemic.

Individual stories such as the beating to death of a young HIV positive woman in South Africa, the speech of 12-year-old Nkosi Johnson at the Durban World AIDS Conference, and high profile civil disobedience from activists have kept HIV/AIDS in South Africa topical, although issues around its political, medical and social character remain unresolved.

HIV in South Africa is the first book to analyse detailed personal, and often very moving, accounts from the South African epidemic, and to link individual experiences to this epidemic's wider social and political context. Drawing on interviews with 37 South Africans affected by HIV, the book attempts to answer the following questions in particular:

- How are people in South Africa finding ways to live with, speak about and resist HIV?
- What resources – from, for instance, religion, politics and medicine – are people drawing on to confront the virus, and how are they changing those resources in the process?
- What is the significance of gender, 'race' and class in HIV's South African context?
- How is South Africa's HIV epidemic affected by the broader African and international politics of HIV and development, by activism, and by the country's apartheid and post-apartheid history?

Using a narrative approach to analyse and understand people's accounts of the HIV epidemic in South Africa, this groundbreaking book also sheds light on epidemics elsewhere in the developing world, especially where there are growing rates of HIV infection. It is essential reading for academics and students of health and social care, as well as healthcare professionals and policy makers.

Corinne Squire is Co-director of the Centre for Narrative Research at the University of East London.

HIV in South Africa

Talking about the big thing

Corinne Squire

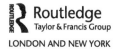

Routledge
Taylor & Francis Group

LONDON AND NEW YORK

First published 2007
by Routledge
2 Park Square, Milton Park, Abingdon, Oxon OX14 4RN

Simultaneously published in the USA and Canada

711 Third Avenue, New York, NY 10017

*Routledge is an imprint of the Taylor & Francis Group, an informa
business*

© 2007 Corinne Squire

Typeset in Times New Roman
by Florence Production Ltd, Stoodleigh, Devon

All rights reserved. No part of this book may be reprinted or
reproduced or utilised in any form or by any electronic, mechanical,
or other means, now known or hereafter invented, including
photocopying and recording, or in any information storage or retrieval
system, without permission in writing from the publishers.

British Library Cataloguing in Publication Data
A catalogue record for this book is available from the British Library

Library of Congress Cataloging-in-Publication Data
Squire, Corinne, 1958–
    HIV in South Africa/Corinne Squire.
        p. cm.
    Includes bibliographical references and index.
    1. Aids (Disease) – South Africa.   2. HIV infections – South
Africa.   I. Title. [DNLM: 1. HIV Infections – epidemiology –
Africa South of the Sahara – Personal Narratives. WC 503.4 HA12
S774h 2007]
    RA643.86.S6S66 2007
    362.196′979200968–dc22   2006102496

ISBN10: 0–415–37209–7 (hbk)
ISBN10: 0–415–37210–0 (pbk)
ISBN10: 0–203–94650–2 (ebk)

ISBN13: 978–0–415–37209–1 (hbk)
ISBN13: 978–0–415–37210–7 (pbk)
ISBN13: 978–0–203–94650–3 (ebk)

Contents

Acknowledgements

I would like to thank the University of East London, particularly the School of Social Sciences, Media and Cultural Studies, for sabbatical support for my research, and all my colleagues, especially Molly Andrews, Maria Tamboukou and Mark Davis, for their encouragement. The University of Cape Town Department of Psychology, especially Don Foster, provided enormous help during my 2001 research and thereafter. The University of KwaZulu-Natal Department of Psychology have been generous hosts and inspiring colleagues; thanks in particular to Yvonne Sliep, Jude Clark and Lindy Wilbraham. Special thanks to Stephanie Kilroe, Elizabeth Kobese, Mandla Majola, Ncumisa Mdinginya, Yolisa Ncethelo and Mary Turok for continuing advice and discussion. Nomvula Zenzile and Sabelo Mazibuko were painstaking and insightful research assistants; Lumka Daniel's work on the research project was invaluable in its creativity and thoughtfulness. Zethu Cakata to provided insightful and careful translation of some transcripts. Neil Turok and Ruby Turok-Squire have been unfailingly tolerant and helpful; I cannot thank them enough. Finally, my greatest debt of respect and gratitude is to the research participants in this study, to whom the book is dedicated.

Announcement

While the majority market for published print books is in the developed world and to developing-world libraries, it is clearly important for books dealing with developing-world topics to be broadly available. Though published in the UK, the book is available free to those with IP addresses on the United Nations Development Programme's Human Development Index of Medium and Low Rankings (see http://hdr.undp.org/hdr2006/pdfs/report/HDR_2006_Tables.pdf), who can apply to the following address: www.ebookstore.tandf.co.uk

All proceeds from the book go to HIV service organisations within South Africa.

Introduction

The many epidemics of HIV

To have been asked to deliver the closing address at this conference, which in a very literal sense concerns itself with matters of life and death, weighs heavily upon me for the gravity of the responsibility placed on one. . . . This is, as I understand it, a gathering of human beings concerned about turning around one of the greatest threats humankind has faced, and certainly the greatest after the end of the great wars of the previous century. . . . Let us not equivocate: a tragedy of unprecedented proportions is unfolding in Africa.

Nelson Mandela, closing speech, International AIDS Conference, Durban, South Africa, 14 July 2000

I need just three years to live so as to tell people about HIV, and I'll try with my friends. Say I tell my friend, 'Girl, have you heard of the big thing?' – that's how they put it – then I would say, 'People, HIV is not something that should make you dislike me.' I would go on to give an example and say, 'I'm like your sister; because I'm also HIV positive, do not treat your sister as if she is no longer a person, she is a person amongst others'.

Busisiwe, Khayelitsha, June 2001

'A person amongst others': people talking about living with HIV

UNAIDS, the joint United Nations programme on HIV/AIDS, declares HIV 'the most globalized epidemic in history' (2004); Nelson Mandela calls it 'one of the greatest threats humankind has faced' (2000). Of approximately 39.5 million HIV positive people in the world, 24.7 million live in sub-Saharan Africa, with about 5.5 million in South Africa (UNAIDS, 2006; UNAIDS/WHO, 2006). UNAIDS (2006) says that the country's AIDS epidemic – 'one of the worst in the world – shows no evidence of a decline'.[1]

This book looks at how people in South Africa have lived with the epidemic over the past ten years. It examines how HIV appears in people's everyday lives, and in popular media, culture, policy and politics in South Africa. In particular, the book tries to answer the questions: How are people in South Africa finding ways to live with, speak about and resist HIV? What resources – from, for instance, religion, politics and medicine – are people drawing on to confront the virus, and how are they changing those resources in the process? What is the significance of class, 'race' and especially gender in HIV's South African context? How is South Africa's HIV epidemic affected by the broader African and international politics of HIV and development, by activism, and by the country's specific pre- and post-colonial and apartheid history?

The book draws on diverse material on HIV from and about South Africa, gathered over the past five years. Much of the material – from academic research, government reports, magazine articles, health education leaflets and television programmes – is in the public domain. However, some, specifically the transcripts and notes from interviews with people infected or affected by HIV, comes from an interview study of people's experiences and expectations of support for living with HIV, which I began in South Africa in 2001, with followup interviews in 2003 and 2004. My findings have much in common with public South African representations of living with HIV, for instance in magazine features or on radio talk shows. They also resonate with the findings of other HIV-related research, both in South Africa and elsewhere. However, my account differs by focusing at length on the representations provided by interviewees themselves, treating these explications as expert accounts. These first-hand accounts are the principal focus of this book. They show South Africans living with the epidemic, drawing on a variety of social and cultural strategies in order to make sense of it, while also situating themselves within the local and global politics of the condition.

In this introductory chapter, I look at some of the factors affecting the South African HIV epidemic. These factors include developed-world neglect; AIDS 'denialism'; the scale of the epidemic; HIV's wide-ranging social and economic effects; HIV's conjunction with the other problems in people's lives such as unemployment, racism, poor health and discrimination and violence against women; the transnational nature of the epidemic; and the effects of South Africa's own specific history and politics. The chapter starts, however, from my research on people's own accounts of how they live with HIV, which forms a crucial part of the book's argument.

I started my South African research after studying, since 1993, the support resources that people in the UK use to live with the epidemic. I was especially interested in the helpful ways of talking about HIV that people developed, often within support groups that brought together people from many different backgrounds who were living with the virus (Squire, 1999, 2003, 2004, 2006). Social support is widely said to help people deal with HIV (Green, 1993). Support groups' useful effects in situations of chronic illness have also frequently been described (Coppa and Boyle, 2003). My experience of HIV support groups, and of the complex and productive ways that people in the UK study talked about support, made me interested in how people in South Africa would use, evaluate and transform their support resources, in what was at the time a situation of very limited medical provision. I wanted to document what kinds of medical, familial and community support structures people living with the epidemic used and developed, how they valued them, and what other kinds of support they wanted. In South Africa in 2001, despite the numbers affected, silence was still a dominant response to HIV, as it had been in the early days of developed-world epidemics, and indeed still is to a large extent. I also wanted to find out how people were managing to talk about HIV, and what resources they were developing to do this.

My UK research spanned pre- and post-antiretroviral treatment eras of the epidemic. Since the mid-1990s, antiretroviral drugs, or ARVs, have been available to most HIV positive people in the developed world who are seriously ill from HIV-related conditions, or whose CD4 white blood cell count – an important indicator of immune strength when you have HIV – is low. ARVs have been relatively successful in these contexts. No one, still in my UK longitudinal study, has died since that time.[2] In 2001, South Africa was on the point of providing mother-to-child transmission – or MTCT – prevention treatment to all pregnant HIV positive women. Some pilot and trial ARV treatment projects were running. However, there was government opposition to extending such treatment on the grounds of expense, ARVs' side-effects, and infrastructural deficits in for instance drug distribution, staff training and patient education. There was also international scepticism about whether people in the developing world could manage ARV treatment, which needs to be taken consistently at specific times in order to work and to avoid resistance developing. That June, USAID Head Andrew Natsios remarked to a journalist that most Africans 'don't know what Western time is . . . and if you say one o'clock in the afternoon, they don't know what you are talking about' (*Boston Globe*, 7 June 2001). I wanted to document people's knowledge of HIV, and their experiences of managing this and other difficult medical treatment situations.

In mid-2001, I and three research assistants, Lumka Daniel, Nomvula Zenzile and Sabelo Mazibuko, conducted interviews with 37 people, 34 of them HIV positive, who lived in townships around Cape Town. We asked them to tell us about what kinds of support they used, liked and wanted for living with HIV. Later, in 2003 and 2004, I returned and spoke to eight of these interviewees again, twice in some cases.

As you might expect, much of what South African interviewees say – as with Busisiwe, quoted at the start of this Introduction – sounds very similar to how people in the developed world talk about HIV. Busisiwe was the pseudonym chosen by a young woman in her 20s, with a child, who had recently lost her second baby because of HIV, and who had experienced serious HIV-related illness herself. Like many interviewees in South Africa and the UK, she talked about dealing with the stigmatisation and uncertainty associated with HIV, trying to live 'positively', and helping others do likewise. Like many interviewees in both countries, Busisiwe said she wanted to be 'a person amongst others', and she talked a great deal about her life beyond the virus – about children, boyfriends, jobs and education. At the same time, Busisiwe's and other South African interviewees' talk about the virus has some very different meanings. Most people living with HIV in South Africa also live with economic, social and educational disadvantage, limited access to effective treatments, and what has been characterised by Mandisa Mbali (2003) and others as 'AIDS denialism' in the political arena.

Three things were notable, for me, about the interviews. First, most interviewees, independently of their contact with formal HIV services, demonstrated high levels of HIV knowledge, strong awareness of what ARV treatment would involve, and considerable skill and determination in accessing and using scarce medical resources, for example, in getting care for children with HIV and other illnesses, successfully undergoing difficult TB treatments, and searching out treatment for opportunistic infections related to HIV. The research, although it came from a small and specific sample, thus made a strong case for the viability of ARV treatment for HIV positive South Africans.

Next, the interviewees used a wide range of strategies for talking about the virus, drawn from western and traditional medicine, religion, politics and popular media such as talk shows. In particular, they mobilised an array of story forms, or genres, to talk about HIV stories, as has happened elsewhere within the pandemic (Carricaburu and Pierret, 1995; Crimp, 1988; Ezzy, 2000; Murphy and Poirier, 1993; Squire, 1999, 2004). These genres often overlapped, and could be subdivided and recombined. However, some, which I look at in later chapters, seemed particularly insistent both in the material, and within the larger context of HIV and popular representations in South Africa. These are, first, a genre of 'speaking out', in which people describe accepting and disclosing their HIV status, usually first within families or support groups, but with plans to extend this disclosure and to build community knowledge and action around HIV. Second, I examine a religious genre of 'conversion' to the belief in HIV as an illness which you can live with, rather than die from; and of commitment to witnessing to this contemporary HIV truth. Third, the book looks at political genres of 'speaking out' that relate to national histories of witnessing and resistance. These forms of representation appeared highly persuasive both for the speakers themselves, and for those of us – researchers and other interviewees – who listened to them. Describing them seemed like a relevant research focus at a time when the many voices of people infected and affected by HIV in the country were starting to gain a hearing.

From our interviewees' commitment to talking about HIV, it appeared that simply talking about the 'big thing', as Busisiwe called it, might make living with it easier. This was the last major finding. In South Africa, silence about or 'othering' HIV (Joffe, 1997) has until recently, been the representational norm. To have some way of representing HIV to yourself and others is therefore, as has been the case elsewhere in the pandemic, a key issue (Galavotti *et al.*, 2001). 'Silence = Death', ACT UP declared in the 1980s in the US (Crimp, 1988), and our interviewees often seemed to agree. At the same time, the *type* of representation is crucial. In 1988, Paula Treichler identified the 'epidemic of signification', much of it stigmatising and discriminatory, growing up around HIV. As Treichler pointed out, the meanings attached to HIV strongly affect how it is lived with: 'language plays a powerful role in producing experience and in certifying that experience as authentic' (1999, 4). Our research participants were very aware that their positive status was shamed and silenced by virtue of its connections with illness, death and transgressive sexualities, and pathologised still further where it was associated with unemployment, poverty, curtailed education and femininity.

By 2001, when our research started, few South Africans had publicly declared themselves HIV positive, but HIV representations in policy, government and popular media were growing rapidly. Politicians, educators, counsellors, activists and our own interviewees all agreed on the importance of finding ways to talk about HIV. For the research participants, the interviews were often a part of that process. Some research participants had spoken out about having HIV to their families and friends. Many were involved with support groups, communities of interest that allowed freedom of HIV speech, and encouraged individual and group programmes of action. For some, talking about HIV in the abstract, listening to conversations about it, or even just seeing TV programmes about it or hearing it talked about on the radio, was a surrogate but also highly meaningful representational repertoire, contributing to what I call a strategy of 'non-disclosing acceptance'.

The shifts in South African HIV institutions and discourses also show that, as elsewhere in the pandemic, the realities around HIV powerfully affect what can be talked about (Ciambrone, 2001; Lown *et al.*, 1993; Monette, 1998). In the absence of treatment, people often see little benefit in getting HIV tested; they may also see little value or possibility in HIV talk. In the neighbourhoods where we conducted research, the growing possibilities of conventional medical treatment for opportunistic infections and for pregnant HIV positive women, and the trial and pilot availability of ARVs, seemed strongly to encourage HIV talk, even among those who could not or did not need to access these treatments.

Talking about HIV is no substitute for material resources. But for many interviewees, as for Busisiwe, it was an important aspect of HIV positive life itself, sometimes even giving a new purpose in that life. Busisiwe had told some family members about her HIV status. However, much of the interview concerned her desire to tell more people about HIV: how you can live with it instead of dying from it; how you can continue to be a 'person amongst others'; and how, if you know enough and are confident enough, you can stop yourself and others from getting it. For Busisiwe and many other interviewees, talking about HIV was a way to build 'interpretive communities' (Plummer, 1995) that would not just support you as an HIV positive person, but would also expand people's knowledge and understanding of HIV generally. These interpretive communities might then become communities of action, helping people live with HIV, fighting for their rights and reducing HIV's spread. At the same time, it is important to note that there are elements of living with HIV that cannot be storied into sense. One example makes its way from Busisiwe's words into the book's subtitle. 'The big thing' is, Busisiwe says, a popular way of referring to HIV without naming it, 'that's what they call it . . .'. In South Africa, HIV continues to generate indirect descriptions – 'the whittling disease', 'wearing the red scarf' (ribbon), 'playing the Lotto', 'TKZ' (a famous band, also named with three letters) – and in our research, 'our disease', 'this torturing thing', 'this awful thing', 'this thing that is spoken about' or simply 'this thing'. This indirectness has been related to traditions of taboo in South African languages (Dowling, n.d.). However, language communities worldwide show similar avoidances when speaking of HIV and other difficult conditions such as cancer (Sontag, 2001). In examining representations of HIV, this book also explores what is unspeakable about the epidemic, and how people deal with these unspoken elements.

The realities and representations of the HIV pandemic are multiple, changing and sometimes contradictory. 'Theorising' the pandemic is usually a matter of creating a working model of one aspect of it. We might, of course, argue that theories are always of this partial, changeable kind. However, HIV's physical mutability, its shifting, transnational epidemics and significations, and the medical uncertainties of managing it, set against its global reach and its potential fatality, dramatise the contingency of its theories. HIV theories of the kind outlined in this book – my own, those of other writers and those of the research participants – are inevitably and appropriately forms of pragmatism, as Cornell West (1989: 211ff.) and Chantal Mouffe (1996) have described it.[3] Pragmatic theories do not try to give complete or permanent explanations. Instead, they aim to provide a framework for understanding, living in, and having effects on contemporary circumstances. At the same time, they have wider commitments to social change. Their particularity is an answer to an ethical responsibility which 'is always unequal to itself. One is never responsible enough' (Derrida, 1995: 51). Theoretical initiatives around HIV need to attain this kind of balance between particularity and generality if they are to address both specific epidemics, and the broad nature and effects of the pandemic.

This is a book written by someone who is British and HIV negative. Being South African and having direct experience of living with the virus would not guarantee a full picture, but it would undoubtedly have allowed richer insights into key questions. There is a great deal of writing coming directly out of the South African epidemic, both from personal and research perspectives (for instance, Abdool Karim and Abdool Karim, 2005; Cameron, 2005a; Campbell, 2003; Kaufman and Lindauer, 2003; Whiteside and Sunter, 2000), but there is room for much more. It is to be hoped that this book will be followed by others that remedy its omissions and superficialities, and that bring into public view more of the knowledge, understanding and engagement of people living with the South African epidemic.

HIV in developed and developing worlds

The South African HIV epidemic has its own controversial history; but that history occurs within the wider 20-year history of an expanding pandemic, and across the economic, political and social divisions between developed and developing worlds. In the developed world today, HIV often seems like an illness of other, poorer people. In the developing world too, it is some-times marginalised as an illness of other countries, or – by the middle classes – of the poor. But migration, and other exchanges and interdependencies within and between nations, mean that HIV is increasingly part of life in all developed- and developing-world countries, across economic and social statuses. The richest and most powerful countries play a determining role, for instance through the Global Fund to Fight AIDS, Tuberculosis and Malaria, in shaping HIV education and treatment throughout the world. Yet, as South Africa's example shows, developing-world countries also effec-tively plan and implement their own HIV policies and campaigns, work with regional and political allies in doing so, and produce powerful movements of HIV-positive and HIV-affected advocates and activists.[4] In the developed world, the commitment and success of such developing-world actions tends to be overlooked, the people behind them reduced to victims or recipients. By exploring representations of HIV in South Africa, in a situation where it is part of everyone's everyday realities, the book aims to bring HIV closer to the realities of readers outside that situation, too.

HIV: normalisation and tragedy

When people in the developed world think about HIV, what usually comes to their minds? Perhaps they, like South Africa's ex-president Nelson Mandela in the quotation that begins this Introduction, think of an 'unfolding tragedy' with which we are all involved. Perhaps they imagine this tragedy as distant and insurmountable, affecting others less fortunate than them-selves, far, far away. They may also recognise in HIV a significant cost, both in humanitarian terms of loss of life, and economically and politically. Since 9/11, developed-world countries have even seen HIV as something of a political threat, contributing to destabilisation through its weakening of economy, state and civil society. At times – especially around World AIDS Day – there is a flurry of media dispatches from the frontlines of HIV prevalence, where high percentages of people are infected. Some empathetic representations appear, focused on the personal stories of individuals living with HIV. Many such reports, however, present HIV in the developing world as a pitiful matter of unsafe sex, victimised women, untreatable illness and inevitable death, all orchestrated by fear, ignorance, resource shortages, poor governance and failures of democracy.

People in the 'developed' world also think of HIV as the fate of those 'socially excluded' within their own societies – drug addicts, sex workers, gay men, refugees and poor people of colour. They may also, at times, think of 'normal' people, just like them, who have HIV – people who are white and middle class, though they may also sometimes be gay. Such 'normal' HIV positive people appear occasionally in popular media, where they are represented as living healthily with HIV, with the help of ARVs if necessary. This normalising representation of HIV, by treating it as more or less irrelevant, erases it.

Thus in the developed world, HIV is increasingly represented in two ways, both of which screen off its wider meanings and realities. First, it appears as a chronic but containable first-world illness. This is an inadequate representation of the social patterns of the first-world epidemic, which as with other health conditions (Krieger *et al.*, 1993; Wilkinson, 2005) are strongly affected by race and gender, and by class. In the US, for instance, 50 per cent of new HIV diagnoses are among African Americans, and the rate of AIDS diagnosis for black women is 23 times that for white women (Centers for Disease Control, 2004). HIV is also not always or easily manageable by ARVs. It continues to be a fatal or seriously health-compromising condition for many in the developed world.

Second, HIV may appear as a tragedy of social exclusion, lived by people who are literally or figuratively exiled from citizenship within developed-world nations, or by people who live elsewhere, 'over there', in foreign, predominantly poor and African contexts. In this viral melodrama, HIV, to use Cindy Patton's metaphor (2002: 47–50), is a 'tropical' condition, spatially organised, emerging from the 'heart of darkness', disseminated via diaspora, always likely to invade or to smuggle itself in secretly to the safe spaces of the developed world (see also Squire, 1997, 2006). This representation, paranoid as well as tragic, tends to exoticise and dehumanise HIV, and also to maintain problematic divisions between developed and developing worlds, and between the 'included' and 'excluded' in the developed world.[5]

What developed-world representations of HIV rarely dwell on is that even if transmission rates fall, effective treatment becomes accessible and a cure or a vaccine is found, the pandemic will continue to grow for the next 20 years at least.[6] It will influence HIV positive people's lives in long-term ways we cannot fully predict, shaping their families' futures, particularly those of their children. And it will pose continuing challenges to many countries' health and social services, economies and governments until at least the middle of this century (Barnett and Whiteside, 2006: 171ff.).

HIV will also become significant in national and local contexts where it has previously been infrequent or overlooked. This expanding 'world' of

HIV significance does not stop at borders. Developed and developing worlds are already connected by migration, tourism, flows of capital, culture, labour and consumption, and international policy and governance. They will become more interlinked, and so will their HIV epidemics. HIV is, as Tony Barnett and Alan Whiteside say, 'the first epidemic of globalisation' (Barnett and Whiteside, 2006: 4).

At present, people in the developed world rarely place themselves on the world HIV scene. We are far from thinking of people with HIV in the framework of common citizenship urged by Busisiwe, in the second quotation that begins this Introduction. The book draws on this interview and others from the HIV support study to provide a picture of South Africa's epidemic that does not resort to pathos, paranoia or normalisation. Instead, it shows people finding strategies to live with the condition in situations of medical underprovision, poverty, social discrimination and international neglect.

HIV and other problems

Even in developing-world countries strongly affected by HIV, there are doubts about its prevalence, physiological effects and treatment. There are concerns, voiced at times for instance by the current South African President, Thabo Mbeki, that many discussions of HIV in the African context are driven by a racism that identifies Africans, African men in particular, with animalistic and uncontrollable sexualities. Such sexualised racism has precedent in colonial addresses to the 'African' body (Butchart, 1988; Fanon, 1986; Gilman, 1985; Manganyi, 1989; Watney, 1990) and to representations of the first 'other' of the HIV pandemic, Haitians (Farmer, 1999). Addresses to HIV also provoke broader political concerns. Perhaps focusing on HIV will cause other important issues such as poverty, racism and general health to be sidelined. High-prevalence countries may become whole-nation patients of western medicine and clients of international pharmaceutical companies. While such arguments can be persuasive, the accompanying tendency to minimise the HIV pandemic means that the specific effects of HIV within societies can be underplayed.

For people with HIV, there may indeed be more pressing issues in their lives than the virus. Struggles against poverty, unemployment, lack of education and other health problems may take precedence.[7] Nevertheless, the virus is a constant part of their lives, presenting particular medical and social problems. In high HIV-prevalence contexts such as South Africa, moreover, HIV becomes everyone's problem. People are likely to be living with HIV within families and neighbourhoods of people who are also affected. Those who are HIV negative or who do not know their status will also have their lives shaped by concerns about HIV transmission and illness.

In these circumstances, the resilient and creative efforts of people living with HIV need to be recognised and learned from, whether they foreground

HIV or, at times, give precedence to other concerns. The book draws on interviewees' formulations of their lives to generate a picture of how HIV is lived within the specific developing-world context of South Africa. That picture overlaps with pictures emerging from some other HIV epidemics, and provides historical echoes and foreshadowings of the pandemic in still other national contexts.

HIV: an overview

HIV's effects

The year 2005 saw 2.8 million HIV-related deaths, bringing the total since 1981 to over 25 million. Beyond this mortality, itself difficult to comprehend, the pandemic has, as Mandela's speech intimated, large and growing social effects. In many high-prevalence African countries, where public sector HIV treatment is only partially available and private treatment is prohibitively costly, HIV is overwhelming health and social services, demoralising their providers, and devastating the manufacturing economy, farming and the educational system. Skilled industrial and agricultural workers, teachers and health workers are dying. Other teachers, doctors and nurses seek employment in the developed world to redress the resource shortages their families face. Life expectancy in high-prevalence African countries such as South Africa and Botswana, has decreased from over 60 in the mid-1990s to around 51 and 35, respectively, today. HIV is also severely eroding social and political structures. Widowed parents, grandparents and older children are increasingly caring for children; there are rising numbers of AIDS orphans.[8]

It is often said that there is no HIV 'pandemic' but rather a range of overlapping epidemics with specific national characteristics, depending on who is affected, levels of HIV prevalence, and the country's economic, social and political state. In South Africa, although the country's economy, infrastructure, health service, media and political institutions are relatively strong, high prevalence, low average incomes and constrained government budgets mean the country has been very powerfully affected. UNAIDS's (2006a) estimate of 5.5 million infected derives from an overall national prevalence of around one-third among pregnant women and 18.8 per cent among all adults, some of the highest rates in sub-Saharan Africa. Despite well-developed public and private health sectors and increasing commitment from government and international programmes, low private health insurance coverage, lack of money to buy private care, and the public sector's continuing partial and patchy delivery of antiretrovirals and other treatments mean that relatively few receive adequate treatment. Nearly 1,000 people die daily. The extent and intractability of the epidemic are such that many now experience 'AIDS fatigue', a term applied both to people overburdened with HIV concerns in their family or at work, and to people who are simply tired of hearing about HIV.

Resisting HIV

In the response to the pandemic over the past 25 years, organisations set up by people infected and affected by HIV have often been the first and most effective actors. Examples include the San Francisco AIDS Project, Gay Men's Health Crisis and ACT UP in the US; the Terrence Higgins Trust in the UK, TASO in Uganda and in South Africa, the Treatment Action Campaign, or TAC.[9] Such organisations were also frequently the first to create international links, as with the International Community of Women Living with HIV/AIDS which reached out from its European beginnings in the mid-1990s to include African and Asian countries, and TASO's mid-1990s collaboration with a parallel Senegalese organisation (Iliffe, 2006: 100; O'Sullivan, 2000).

International non-governmental organisations such as the World Health Organisation (WHO) were slow to take HIV in the developing world seriously (Iliffe, 2006: 68), at least until 1986; the first WHO declared World AIDS Day was in 1988. Charity non-governmental organisations (NGOs) such as the Red Cross and Médecins sans Frontières (MSF) have been leaders in HIV education and treatment; MSF started ARV programmes in 2000 and by 2005 had 31 programmes in 16 countries, mostly free of charge (Médecins sans Frontières, 2005). Other NGOs such as Oxfam and Christian Aid routinely address HIV within their broader remits.

HIV is, however, as UNAIDS notes, 'unique' in being both 'an emergency *and* a long-term development issue' (2004: 15). It demands enormous resources to address the health crisis it has precipitated, while also needing to be aligned with more general development policies. Consequently, UN-related organisations, such as the WHO, the UN, through its HIV and AIDS programme, UNAIDS, UNESCO and UNICEF, and the World Bank, have become more and more significant in HIV initiatives. The tradition in international public health work of limiting and stabilising epidemics, followed by efforts to remove them as endemic conditions from populations, is accompanied in the case of HIV by serious attention to the long-term effects of the pandemic on social and economic structures.

Private foundations and charities have made substantial worldwide contributions to HIV education and treatment projects, from the Gates and Merck Foundations funding Botswana's ARV treatment programme to the Elton John AIDS Foundation, which has supported HIV prevention and education projects worldwide since 1992, and the Clinton Foundation's recent brokering of agreements to provide cheaper first- and second-line antiretroviral treatment to low- and middle-income countries. In South Africa, a number of private companies such as De Beers and Anglo-American have provided ARVs as well as other treatment and prevention services for their workers (Department of Health, 2006) for several years, considerably sooner than the public provision of antiretroviral treatment – though numbers benefiting remain small.

It is frequently argued that the seriousness and consistency of government responses have a determining effect on the progress of HIV epidemics (Barnett and Whiteside, 2006). National-level responses have been extremely variable. President Reagan famously did not utter the word 'AIDS' until 1985, four years into the US epidemic. South Africa produced its first five-year plan for dealing with the epidemic in 2000. Its Comprehensive HIV/AIDS Care Management and Treatment Plan was not ratified until the end of 2003. There have been many occasions on which the government's perceived ambivalence about the causes and treatment of HIV has gained worldwide attention, and its delivery of HIV treatment continues to be sceptically assessed. Other governments' responses have been, by contrast, committed and consistent. The government of Thailand instituted a blanket AIDS education and prevention programme in 1991 and provided treatment for pregnant HIV positive women from 1999. Uganda began its national response in 1992 and started providing ARVs in 1998. Botswana pursued a full ARV treatment programme from 2002, working with private corporations. There are difficulties – for instance, with Uganda's and Botswana's still-incomplete levels of ARV coverage and medical staffing. In Uganda, erratic drug supplies, the costs of HIV care and the abstention from sex message now required by some US-funded ARV programmes remain problematic. Botswana's early reliance on privately funded programmes was controversial. Yet like Thailand, these countries engaged seriously with HIV at all levels, led by presidents and governments committed to the issue.[10]

Against the pandemic's undeniable and large-scale crises, local, national and international education and treatment programmes are slowly and unevenly getting to grips with the pandemic, trying to stabilise infection rates, and extend medical treatment to new populations and conditions and address the social and economic relations within which prevention must work (Barnett and Whiteside, 2006: 78ff.). Despite condom availability estimated to be around 50 per cent of what low- and middle-income countries need (Population Action International, 2006), and the mixed success of programmes using the Abstain, Be Faithful, Condomise or ABC agenda, introduced in the 1990s, new infections are slowing or declining in many countries, particularly among young urban people in heavily affected African countries. International aid programmes, alongside developing-world countries' own financial commitments to expanding treatment, meant that over 1.3 million people were receiving HIV treatment in sub-Saharan Africa by the end of 2006, about 28 per cent of those estimated to need it (World Health Organisation, 2007). These small numbers are still an important step, begun under the '3 by 5' initiative of the United Nations' AIDS programme, UNAIDS, and the World Health Organisation. This optimistic plan aimed to get 3 million people ARV treatment by the end of 2005, a goal met a year late.[11] Treatment expansion initiatives are still beset with funding uncertainties. Programmes funded by the US President's Emergency Plan for AIDS Relief, PEPFAR, provide the most cutting-edge and extensive care, but are dangerously compromised by PEPFAR's ties to large, mostly US-based pharmaceutical companies, and by its socially conservative agenda, promoting abstention from sex, and restricting condom education and needle exchanges. Brazil, indeed, refused this funding on the grounds that it compromised provision of HIV services to sex workers. Political commitment to universal treatment is also ambivalent. The G8 and, later, the African Union's follow-on to '3 by 5', a commitment to working across Africa for 25 per cent HIV prevalence reduction and 80 per cent HIV service coverage, including ARVs, by 2010 (African Union, 2006), has not been supported subsequently at the UN, or by all the countries involved.

More generally, initiatives that range from neighbourhood education and homecare groups, 'community-based organisations' or CBOs, through national social and health service provision to international non-governmental projects, try to address the stigmatisation, fear and neglect that often accompanies the pandemic, and to support people in staying negative and in living healthily with HIV. Such initiatives can be short-term and tokenist. They may leach scarce resources into local HIV services and at higher levels into an increasingly bureaucratised worldwide HIV 'industry'. However, where these initiatives address HIV in ways that integrate it with other developing-world concerns, they can work to strengthen general health, education, skills and income generation capacity, and to combat gender inequity and gender violence, as well as addressing HIV prevention and treatment.

The pandemic itself shifts, even as communities and agencies try to engage with it. In 2004, UNAIDS proclaimed the 'Next Agenda', which, while it continues to promote condom use, education and destigmatisation, declares that the 'veil of silence' has been lifted. It focuses on providing ARV treatment, and planning for economic and social renewal in the face of the large-scale loss of workers from many employment sectors; high numbers of HIV orphans, now estimated at 12 million in sub-Saharan Africa; and a 'new generation' of people at risk of becoming HIV infected, who do not remember the early days of the pandemic. 2005's UNAIDS 'Three Ones' agreement institutes nationally agreed frameworks for programmes around HIV; their coordination; and their monitoring and evaluation (UNAIDS, 2005), all of which are seen as essential for long-term programmes of treatment and renewal. International agencies also increasingly try to address HIV alongside other economic and health issues, most notably through the Global Fund to fight AIDS, Tuberculosis and Malaria.[12]

In South Africa, over the past decade of the epidemic, a great deal has changed. HIV has moved from being almost unmentionable to being spoken about everywhere – sometimes with counterproductive ubiquity – on radio talk shows and TV dramas, in all medical settings, in education institutions from primary school on, in workplaces, in bars and in clubs. Awareness seemed to grow from a series of incidents highlighted in the media; from dramatic increases in popular representations of HIV since the late 1990s;

and from the activities of a large number of local and national community-based, NGO and government organisations.

In 1998, a young Durban woman, Gugu Dlamini, was beaten to death after she declared her HIV positive status. In 2000, Nkosi Johnson, an 11-year-old HIV positive boy, spoke movingly at the International AIDS Conference about his life and the lives of other infected people in South Africa (Johnson, 2001). These events were widely covered in the media, internationally as well as in South Africa, and in the interview study we did in 2001 they were mentioned by research participants as key moments in their own under-standing of the epidemic. More recently, a string of public figures' dis-closures of their own or family members' HIV positive status; struggles for treatment for pregnant HIV positive women, and for ARVs generally; the claims of a variety of practitioners outside conventional medicine to be able to cure HIV; and the high profile trial of Vice-President Jacob Zuma, acquitted of the rape of an HIV positive woman, have all precipitated national discussions about the epidemic and how to address it.

With more representation came increased organisation and action. The *Soul City* NGO began broadcasting TV and radio shows in the mid-1990s and has become a continent-wide model of HIV 'edutainment' (Papa *et al.*, 2001). The government has supported a youth education and prevention programme, loveLife, since 1999 and between 2002 and 2006, an education and health promotion programme, Khomanani, or Caring Together, which helped people to take action around HIV under the slogan, 'to Care; to Talk; to Test; to Condomise'.[13] At the start of 2004, government began a rollout of ARVs to clinics throughout the country. Some 325,000 people now receive ARVs, around 32 per cent of those who need it (World Health Organisation, 2007) – well below WHO targets, but still about 10 times as many as were receiving treatment in 2003. Many people are involved as voluntary and paid educators and activists, sometimes in local neighbour-hoods, setting up their own support or campaigning groups, sometimes within larger HIV organisations or other CBOs. South African HIV activists have a long history dating back to the early 1990s. Their post-2000 attempts to expand treatment through the Treatment Action Campaign, taking the government as well as pharmaceutical companies to court and mounting civil disobedience campaigns, are perhaps their most internationally recognised aspect. However, community-based campaigns are much more wide-ranging than this, including, for instance, efforts to build local resistance to violence against women, setting up income generation projects for people affected by the virus, and providing food, clothes and childcare for families stretched to breaking point by HIV illness and deaths.

South Africans' awareness of the epidemic and their formulations of ways to deal with it have, then, grown dramatically. While this book cannot give a full picture of these engagements, it aims to provide some account of them, and in particular to describe some of the new forms of representation that people with HIV have developed to build communities of support for themselves and for others affected by the virus. In the case of South Africa, such communities are coming, over time, to include the entire nation.

The HIV pandemic is not just differentiated into national epidemics. HIV is also lived as different epidemics, according to people's very different social positions. The next section of this Introduction explores some of those differences.

A gendered pandemic

HIV has had particularly powerful consequences for women. As UN Secretary-General Kofi Annan said on International Women's Day, 2004, 'society pays many times over the deadly price of the impact on women of AIDS' (Annan, 2004). New infections, particularly among young women, have plateaued or are falling in several sub-Saharan African countries, albeit at a high level. Yet in many high-prevalence countries, women, particularly young women, continue to have higher infection rates. Around 60 per cent of all cases in sub-Saharan Africa are among women. In badly affected countries such as South Africa, at least three times as many 15- to 24-year-old women as men are infected (UNAIDS 2006). In the province of KwaZulu-Natal, where overall prevalence is highest, 15.4 per cent of black African girls aged 15 to 19 and only 2.58 per cent of black African boys of those ages were HIV positive in an early-2000s survey (Morrell *et al.*, 2002). Women are more physiologically susceptible to infection through heterosexual sex; more socially vulnerable to unsafe behaviours in situations of violence, coercion and economic deprivation (Dunkle *et al.*, 2004); more stigmatised as responsible for getting and transmitting HIV, particularly through 'promiscuity'; and less likely to access HIV services except those provided perinatally. Women and girls are more likely to be carers for other HIV-infected family members and orphaned children, and to lose access to education and employment through this labour, as well as their own HIV illness – though men and boys may be disadvantaged in these ways too. Family income loss through AIDS may also disproportionately reduce girls' schooling.

Clinicians, policy-makers and politicians neglected gendered aspects of the pandemic early on, particularly in developed-world epidemics concentrated among gay men and largely male drug users.[14] The 'feminisation' of the developing-world pandemic meant that women were at the forefront of many local and national HIV programmes. Still, gender was not emphasised in UN HIV work until 2001. Since then it has been a growing priority. The XV World AIDS Congress, held in Bangkok in July 2004, had 'Access for All' as its theme, one chosen to foreground women's concerns within a framework of universal human rights. UNAIDS declared 2004 the year of 'Women Girls HIV and AIDS' and launched the Global Coalition on Women and AIDS, a collaboration of the UN, the public sector, civil society and academics. Such international agencies are also recognising women's specific requirements within the pandemic. Acknowledging the gendered limitations of the Abstain, Be Faithful, Condomise, or ABC programme, for instance, they are exploring alternative strategies such as microbicides and the female condom, both of which are positively regarded by women and men in many high-prevalence African countries and can strengthen women's sexual decision-making power.

In South Africa, mother-to-child-transmission prevention treatment – commonly referred to as MTCT – is highly effective. Involving voluntary HIV counselling and testing (VCT), a brief period of antiretroviral medication and – where safe water supplies are available – the provision of infant formula, it has been available since 2001. It is now claimed to reach 79 per cent of pregnant HIV positive women (Department of Health, 2006). As in many other high-prevalence countries, MTCT is the most accessible antiretroviral treatment. Women's experiences with it make them highly aware of HIV issues and prepare them for ARV treatment. South Africa also makes strong constitutional and policy commitments to women's equality and rights, particularly in the context of what is often referred to as another and related 'epidemic' of gender violence. Locally and nationally, women are leading figures in many HIV organisations, addressing the links between gender violence and HIV (Dunkle *et al.*, 2004), opposing stigmatisation and calling for different ways of thinking and talking about HIV and sex. However, HIV public information campaigns have tended not to address gender inequities. HIV programmes in schools are slow to address gender issues, including violence (Moletsane *et al.*, 2002). Community HIV programmes are often jeopardised by the larger socioeconomic formations around gender within which their constituents live (Campbell, 2003).

This book is concerned with men's *and* women's experiences of and responses to HIV, but South African women's vulnerabilities to HIV, alongside their strategies for addressing it, are recurring issues. Women constituted the majority of participants in the 2001–4 research. Many were very keen to take part in a project where they could talk, openly but confidentially, about living with HIV. The male participants, however, were also very engaged in the research and were highly aware of gendered issues in the epidemic, such as men's coercion and health risk-taking in heterosexual relations, and men's lesser likelihood of coming forward for treatment and support. In this awareness, they foreshadowed the growing current concern to make the gendered aspects of HIV priorities for men as well as women.

The economics of living with HIV

Inevitably, economic divisions also have effects on the way HIV is lived with. Developing-world countries contain small, economically privileged groups who can buy the HIV treatment that is inaccessible to their fellow citizens. In first-world countries such as the US, which despite their higher average incomes are also economically divided, HIV treatment success is again financially stratified, and poorer social groups are disproportionately affected.

In South Africa, HIV is not only a disease of poor people. As in other high-prevalence countries, large numbers of urban and mobile young people, and the educated professional classes including teachers, health workers and businesspeople – both groups that index development – are heavily affected (Nelson Mandela Foundation/HSRC, 2002). While striving for growth, investment and social justice, the country is facing an AIDS-related real decline in gross domestic product that a UNAIDS estimate puts at 17 per cent by 2010 (Rosen *et al.*, 2004). HIV also makes large and growing claims on health and social service funding. These claims cannot all be met. People who expected a reasonable standard of living, post-apartheid, are being made poor by their own or family members' illness, both through loss of income and through having to pay for prescription and non-prescription medications, special foods and other provisions.

Unemployment in South Africa is high: a conservative estimate is 27 per cent (Statistics South Africa, 2005). For people who are unemployed or working in the informal economy, HIV means even less chance of earning. It increases the numbers depending on social benefits, particularly pensions, disability and care-dependency grants, which support far more than the 10 million people to whom they are issued.[15] Benefit recipients such as those issued to grandparents, those who are ill themselves, or those looking after orphaned children are often the only family members with a steady income. With unemployment rates well above 50 per cent in some high HIV prevalence areas and among younger people, and with uncertain health, there are few opportunities for HIV positive people to earn a living wage. Without it, buying healthy food to maintain immunity is difficult. As people start to use ARVs, they must also, as has happened in developed-world epidemics, trade the benefits of working against the possibility of work compromising their health, and the problem of having to renegotiate benefits if their health deteriorates.

The racialisation of HIV

Experiences of the epidemic – from infection rates to forms of treatment – are highly differentiated by 'race' and ethnicity (Gilbert and Wright, 2002). HIV's racialisation is particularly salient in South Africa, given the country's history of apartheid and white-minority government, which constructed a hierarchy of racialised population groups with stratified access to education, housing, employment and health services. The democratically elected governments of the post-1994 period have tried to undo this legacy and to provide good quality services for all, but racism remains alive though often unspoken discourse in all areas of society, including around HIV – especially since the virus is currently most common among the 80 per cent of the population that is black African, and least common among the 9.3 per cent white South Africans.[16] Among young people, in the most high-prevalence area of the country, ten times as many black Africans as whites or Indians are affected (Morrell *et al.*, 2002). Figures of this kind have large margins of error. The most recent South African Household Survey that recorded racialised categories had only a 55 per cent response rate (responding was lowest among whites and Indians). It registered an HIV prevalence of 10.8 per cent – 8 per cent lower than the UNAIDS estimate. Among whites, 0.6 per cent were HIV positive, among Indians, 1.6 per cent were HIV positive. HIV rates among black Africans were 13.3 per cent, and among mixed race or coloured people, 1.9 per cent (Shisana *et al.*, 2005). Despite the data's uncertainties, there are clearly some significant differences, within the epidemic, between these historically defined groups.

This book cannot hope to map the political complexities of contemporary South Africa in the arena of 'race', especially as it is written by a white non-South African. However, it is important to remember throughout that this epidemic is occurring in the very specific historical aftermath of a system of government based on racialised and racist ideologies and practices, and the struggle against them.

Social and cultural formations

The far-reaching effects of the South African epidemic will be social and cultural, as well as economic. Education is curtailed through teachers' deaths; through wage loss, which means less money for school fees; and through children's own illnesses and their work as carers for family members with HIV and HIV orphans. There are around 1.2 million AIDS orphans (UNAIDS, 2006), HIV negative or living with HIV, whose future lives will be heavily affected by their childhoods in crisis. Foster care has proved inadequate and child-headed households unworkable; despite general public opposition to the idea, the government is considering new orphanages (Webb, 2006). A second, 'post-treatment' epidemic is developing of people dealing with the psychological and physiological effects of lifelong dependence on drugs. Everyone in South Africa lives continuously with the issues of HIV illness and transmission: at work, with friends, in your family and in relationships. In a nation remaking itself after a long and successful struggle against oppressive and discriminatory government, and trying to implement its radical new constitution's commitment to good health care, a high standard of living and opportunities for all, this is an onerous and unexpected burden to have to take on.

Many cultural formations impact people living with HIV, but perhaps the most salient across different national epidemics are those of religion. The significance of religious institutions and leaders in shaping responses to the epidemic can compare to that of governments. Local structures of faith – what is said and done at religious gatherings, or when individuals talk to their pastor, iman or priest – powerfully affect the lives of people living with or affected by the virus. In developing-world countries, religion often has a strong and generalised presence in social and cultural life. In South Africa, its authority also stems from its place within the anti-apartheid liberation struggle. This book will not be able to review fully South African religious perspectives on the epidemic, but it does aim to demonstrate the power of religious institutions and discourse to affect people's HIV positive lives by providing or denying ethical and practical resources for them.

Intranational, national and transnational epidemics

South Africa's HIV epidemic has, like that of several of its neighbours such as Botswana and Swaziland, a specific and dramatic history. Rates of HIV were low in the 1990s, but increased rapidly during that decade, resulting in a generalised, high-prevalence epidemic by the end of the millennium (Abdool Karim and Abdool Karim, 2002), which is continuing with high annual rates of new infections and deaths. Within South Africa, however, rates vary between genders, ages and racialised groups, as we have seen, and also between the nine provinces. Among antenatal clinic attenders in KwaZulu-Natal in 2005, 39.1 per cent tested positive, compared to 18.1 per cent in the Northern Cape and 15.7 per cent in the Western Cape, where I conducted my research (Department of Health, 2005a). Again, such figures pose difficulties of interpretation. Black Africans, currently most affected by HIV, comprise only 27 per cent of the Western Cape population (Statistics South Africa, 2001). KwaZulu-Natal clinics tend to be located near transport routes, where HIV rates are higher. Women who attend antenatal clinics are not representative of all women, let alone the whole population. UNAIDS's prevalence figures use these data alongside the HSRC Household Survey and other surveys, to arrive at their much lower 18.8 per cent prevalence estimate. Moreover, the percentage of HIV positive women attending KwaZulu-Natal clinics is now falling, whereas the percentage in other provinces – except for Gauteng, the most urbanised – is rising. Rates may rise not only because HIV infection is increasing, but because more women who know or suspect they are positive attend clinics now that MTCT is available, giving them a good chance of having an HIV negative child. Rates may also appear to fall in provinces where the epidemic has been established longer, because HIV positive women are less fertile – or are ill, or dying – rather than because fewer women are HIV positive. Despite these complexities, and notwithstanding overall extremely high levels of HIV infection, the figures do indicate a geographical variability in the epidemic that has its own complex local and national causes and consequences.

While HIV epidemics take specific national and intranational forms, they also increasingly display transnational characteristics. Extensive population shifts as migrants, refugees and tourists move within and between developing and overdeveloped worlds affect their character. In the UK, for example, new infections among men who have sex with men remain high, and rates are rising among heterosexuals. However, two-thirds of those who are HIV positive in the UK were infected heterosexually, three-quarters of these in Africa; 63 per cent of these heterosexual infections are among women (Health Protection Agency, 2005). South Africa's epidemic, apart from being inflected by internal migration, is also now characterised by migration from nearby countries, particularly Zimbabwe: around 1.2 million Zimbabweans are estimated to be living in the country.[17] At the same time, many other forms of transnational exchange occur that are highly relevant for HIV. Large volumes of financial and other forms of support are sent from developed to developing-world countries by migrants and refugees. International organisations such as the Global Fund to Fight AIDS, Tuberculosis and Malaria deliver first-world resources to developing-world epidemics. HIV research itself operates in an integrated, cross-national way, investigating the effects of ARV treatment or of microbicidal HIV prevention, for instance, across African countries.[18] Within a postcolonial political landscape, these transnational links are not all of the same kind. Those affecting research, and education and treatment funding, for example, are largely dictated by first-world countries and international NGOs. By contrast, within Africa, South Africa's relative prosperity and stability yields its own sphere of influence.

South Africa's epidemic must, finally, be seen in the context of the country's unique political profile. The country is a political leader on the African continent. Internationally, its successful struggle against apartheid and for democracy is much admired. This visibility continually impacts its HIV research and policy, its education and treatment programmes, and South Africans' political and personal views on the pandemic. The epidemic and how it is addressed has potentially enormous significance for South Africa itself, but also for the rest of Africa and other parts of the developing world facing their own HIV epidemics and observing South Africa's response to this large and unpredicted crisis. The world outside South Africa is also interested in how the country is managing the difficult yet hopeful task of building a post-apartheid nation, and in how that task encompasses the HIV epidemic. The 'new' South Africa pursues political transformation, social change, economic development and a culture of accountability with tolerance – often emblematised, for the rest of the world, in the Truth and Reconciliation Commission. It is also constructing transnational roles for itself within southern Africa, and across Africa and the developing world, through for instance the African Union, the New Partnership for Africa's Development (NEPAD) and the World Trade Organisation. Is the HIV epidemic an insurmountable obstacle to this programme or can it be included within it?

The South African HIV epidemic's relations with gender, economics, 'race', social and cultural structures, and its intranational, national and transnational characteristics, may not be foregrounded when people in South Africa discuss their own relationship to HIV, but they form the context within which they must deal with their own or others' infection. This is of course a context very different from that in low-HIV prevalence communities, nations and areas of the world, where the fabric of social and cultural life is at least potentially able to 'mend' around tears caused by HIV epidemics. The situation also differs dramatically from that in high-income countries, where funding levels allow health, social services and the voluntary sector to address HIV issues relatively effectively, even when they serve high-prevalence communities. The book emphasises South Africans' innovative and positive engagements with the problems of HIV, but it is important to situate these achievements within a realistic appraisal of the epidemic's drastic effects. The next chapter explores this juxtaposition between national and regional crisis, and responses to it within a general history of the South African epidemic.

1 HIV in South Africa

Global, local and historical realities

When I was first tested in 1997 . . . I didn't think anything, you know the problem was that, I just ignore it, ignore the point of HIV. And then we had that problem, we had the problem of, of us the people in South Africa . . . We took the HIV issue light and we compare it to . . . the countries like, like America . . . we didn't compare it to in South Africa that HIV can be here you know. I took it light and I ignore it just like that, 'No, this is not a truth that I'm HIV positive.' I just ignore it, and the doctor didn't give me the guidelines, how to live with HIV, I must do this and this.

Michael, Khayelitsha, June 2001

I want people to understand about AIDS – to be careful and respect AIDS. You can't get Aids if you touch, hug, kiss, hold hands with someone who is infected. Care for us and accept us – we are all human beings.
We are normal. We have hands. We have feet.
We can walk, we can talk, we have needs just like everyone else – don't be afraid of us – we are all the same!

Nkosi Johnson, speaking at the 2000 International AIDS Conference,
Durban, South Africa (Johnson, 2001)

I have said that the government will continue with its programme on this matter of HIV and AIDS and I have nothing more to add to it.

President Thabo Mbeki, in discussion following
questions in the National Assembly, 21 October
2004, *Cape Times*, 22 October 2004

HIV in the world

In 2003, I walked into a pharmacy in Cape Town's bustling train station and bought a bottle of herbal tonic called Africa's Solution. It was not like any other remedy I'd seen. From street sellers, you could buy locally made tonics that claimed to have good effects on HIV; some of our interviewees had tried these. In pharmacies, you could buy herbal remedies, soberly packaged, advertising a wide range of healthful properties; some interviewees used these, too. Africa's Solution was different. Red, green, black and gold, like a brightly coloured African flag, it promised the indigenous answer that President Mbeki and many others hoped for. It claimed to help 'tiredness and fatigue . . . chronic chest, perspiration at night, swollen glands', all possible symptoms of HIV. A picture of a whiskery African potato, the mainstay of health minister Manto Tshabalala-Msimang's nutritional advice for people with HIV, adorned the label. Retailing at R39.95 a bottle – then nearly one-tenth of the monthly disability allowance – few people living with HIV could afford Africa's Solution, but many would try anyway. It had a pleasant, vegetably taste, and lasted two years in my fridge before fermenting.

In 2004, Africa's Solution became famous. A Dutch-national nurse and her mother, Tine and Nelly van der Maas, promoted the use of the tonic alongside food supplements and fresh fruit and vegetables, as obviating the need for antiretrovirals. They continue to claim that their work in various South African provinces has shown the regime's good effects in raising numbers of CD4 white blood cells and lowering viral load, the amount of HIV in the blood.[1] But no independent research has backed these claims. There is speculation that the van der Maases get a cut from the sales of Africa's Solution. In 2005 two public figures, the Johannesburg DJ Fana Khaba in 2004 and Nosipho Bhengu (daughter of Ruth Bhenghu, a promi-nent ANC MP) died of AIDS while promoting the van der Maas regime (McGregor, 2006; Treatment Action Campaign, 2006). Khaba, indeed, abandoned antiretrovirals for the regime. One explanation for these and other HIV positive people's turning to Africa's Solution is that it may have some beneficial effects. A programme of nutrition-rich foods and supplements can improve health, at least initially. The van der Maas's patients are often, like many other people in South Africa, malnourished, with multiple health problems. Moreover, antiretrovirals are not always easy medications to take, and adjusting to lifelong medication is difficult. But South Africa's specific history of HIV, apartheid and postcolonialism is also what has given Africa's Solution – a South African product, promoted by two commonsense women with no airs of medical expertise or NGO graces – its prominent, though contested, place.

This chapter examines theories of the beginning and spread of HIV in South Africa, and describes medical, governmental, activist and popular responses to it. Such situating of the epidemic is not a formal exercise. The extent, causes and history of HIV are continually talked about in South Africa, not just among politicians and intellectuals, but among ordinary people. You often hear people asking, 'How did HIV get to be such an enormous problem here?', expressing bewilderment in the face of this generalised and high-level epidemic, but also offering answers.

Many of the interviewees in our research project were deeply concerned about these issues. Not only must they live with a potentially fatal condition in a severely under-resourced context; it seemed they must share this circumstance with a high proportion of their fellow citizens. They must also imagine, not a post-apartheid national future of education and development, 'a better life for all', as the 1994 election slogan had it, but a future of illness, bereavement and social decline. Such experiences are hard to live with (Odets, 1995); they impel you to try to understand them. For South Africans affected by HIV – that is, everyone in the country – talking about the 'big thing' does not, therefore, simply involve personal concerns, but also considerations of larger issues. Such wide-ranging talk helps build theories of the global as well as local realities of HIV – theories that can help people in their efforts to live with the virus.

The fastest-growing HIV epidemics in the world are currently in Eastern Europe and Asia (UNAIDS, 2006), but prevalence in these epidemics does not reach southern African levels. India now has more cases of HIV than South Africa; again, the virus's prevalence in southern Africa is much greater. In some west and central African countries, HIV prevalence seems fairly stable at between 5 per cent and 10 per cent (UNAIDS, 2006). In a few east and central African countries such as Uganda and Tanzania, prevalence has fallen, with HIV stabilising at relatively low levels (Iliffe, 2006; Lutambi, 2005). In southern African countries, however, while new infections are plateauing, prevalence may not peak until around 2013 (Johnson and Dorrington, 2006; Lutambi, 2005). In these countries, HIV also dispro-portionately affects younger people (MacPhail *et al.*, 2002), as opposed to Tanzania for instance where HIV prevalence is more evenly distributed across age groups (Favot *et al.*, 1997). Although South Africa spends more than most middle-income nations on health as a percentage of gross domestic product – 5 per cent in 1990, 8 per cent in 2003 – HIV also spread faster there than in low-income Tanzania. Botswana, Swaziland, Lesotho and Zimbabwe have higher HIV prevalences than South Africa, and a similar chronological profile of an epidemic that rapidly expanded in the 1990s, and that now affects the whole nation; but their epidemics involve lower absolute numbers.[2]

Achieving democracy after a 50-year struggle, only to face a new national struggle that must be conducted on the very different grounds of medicine and social relationships, also puts South Africa in a unique position.[3] The rest of this chapter tries to address debates about the South African epidemic through examining, first, explanations of how the virus arose and how it spread in Africa; and second, South African responses to HIV.

Explaining the pandemic

Explanations of the South African epidemic take three forms. First, there are widely accepted, research-derived forms, as presented by international organisations, medical authorities and NGOs; second, some popularised, implicitly racist variants; and third, explanations that oppose this second type, and that have developed in some high HIV-prevalence areas. I shall draw briefly on our 2001–4 interviews to illustrate how explanations of the epidemic appear within people's accounts of HIV and can affect their ways of living with the virus.

The accepted chronology of the pandemic begins in 1981, when the US Centers for Disease Control published the first reports of unusually high incidences of rare kinds of pneumonia, skin cancer and cytomegalovirus infection – all pointing to problems in immune system functioning – among gay men in California and New York (Friedman *et al.*, 1981). This 'Gay Related Immune Deficiency Syndrome' or 'GRIDS' was renamed 'AIDS' the next year, and the HIV virus underlying the symptoms isolated in 1983.[4] However, it is probable that HIV has a much longer and more dispersed existence in humans, involving long-term low levels of infection. HIV has been isolated from a 1959 plasma sample, but may have been around in humans since the 1930s within Africa, moving to the US and then Haiti in the late 1970s.[5] It is thought to derive from west and west-central African monkey retroviruses that crossed species and hybridised in chimpanzees, forming Simian Immunodeficiency Virus, SIV. This virus was then transmitted to other chimps and other species, notably humans (Keele *et al.*, 2006). Such interspecies transmission could have happened through blood-to-blood transmission during hunting – much as earlier versions of the virus may have moved from monkeys to chimps. Many viruses, bacteria and other disease-causing entities cross species – most notably at present, avian flu. Some, such as BSE and salmonella, do so through meat consumption. Other monkey viruses are also found in humans where monkeys are eaten.

When we encounter nonhuman viruses, we are usually unaffected, or we fight them off. Occasionally, however, SIV would have mutated in humans into a more resistant form – HIV. Supporting this account, contemporary HIV and related simian viruses have many strains and high mutation rates (Goulder and Watkins, 2004) – again, like many other disease-causing entities such as flu viruses.

Why do the origins of HIV matter so much for the ways in which people now live with it? In the Introduction, I described the 'epidemic of signification' (Treichler, 1988) that has consistently surrounded the virus. This 'epidemic' has also taken in HIV's. African beginning, which is often discussed in the west in ways that repeat colonial mythologies of the animalistic 'African' mentioned in the Introduction (Chirimuuta and Chirimuuta, 1989).[6] In such mythological accounts, there is a liminal place in 'the heart of Africa' where boundaries between humans, and between humans and animals, break down. Responding to these racist constructions, oppositional theories of HIV's origin have often developed in Haiti, for instance, as well as in South Africa. Some such theories, like the one described at the beginning of this chapter by Michael, the pseudonym of one of our interviewees, identify HIV with western promiscuity, intravenous drug use and male homosexuality. Similarly, in Paul Farmer's study of HIV and TB in rural Haiti, people reported HIV's place of origin as the US or the US-influenced city (1999: 161). Other oppositional theories ascribe HIV to a CIA programme of biological warfare against Africa, perhaps performed through vaccinations. Where, as in many places in the developing world, medical interventions focus largely on childhood immunisation, to suspect such a connection makes some sense. Immunisations' links to other health problems are indeed often a public concern, as in western debates over the relation between the MMR vaccination and autism, or recent fears in northern Nigeria that polio vaccine contained either HIV or an anti-fertility agent (World Health Organisation, 2004). Developing-world countries also have a long history of being the subjects of unethical medical experimentation; this shaped many Haitians' initial understandings of HIV (Farmer, 1999: 164). The 40-year Tuskegee experiment, beginning in 1932 and involving 399 African–American men deliberately not told of or treated for their syphilis diagnosis (Jones, 1993) is often cited in such accounts to emblematise western science's racism. HIV medication and vaccine trials, conducted in situations where resource shortages compromise the meaning of 'consent', often seem to be engaged in similarly unethical endeavours. Such trials frequently, for example, involve placebos (Milford *et al.*, 2006; see also Abdool Karim, 1998) – a procedure successfully fought in western ARV research by activists in the early 1990s, and in developing-world mother to child HIV transmission (MTCT) prevention treatment research in the late 1990s. Developing countries are also concerned about pharmaceutical companies' power, in situations of low government provision and regulation. More broadly, racialised economic and social disadvantage certainly play a part in the South African HIV epidemic, as they do in high HIV-prevalence urban African American communities (Lown *et al.*, 1993), and in Haiti (Farmer, 1999). In South Africa, moreover, HIV raises for many the memory of apartheid-era plans for biological weapons (Robins, 2004).

Another oppositional account of the HIV epidemic sees the virus as fairly harmless, or as relatively low in prevalence – a position sometimes supported by contradictory prevalence figures like those explored in the Introduction. In this account, HIV is said to operate as a western pretext for expanding pharmaceutical markets, with ARVs the toxic agents of postcolonial medicalisation and economic subjugation. The causes of 'HIV' symptoms are said to be poverty and simpler, less profitable diseases. From this perspective, HIV may also be viewed as a western excuse for reducing Africa's population through condomisation. WHO and other international contraceptive campaigns, the developed-world discourse of developing-world overpopulation, and western pathologisations of 'African' sexualities can render such an account plausible.[7] Moreover, nonwhite South Africans have already experienced apartheid programmes of sexualised as well as racialised control.

Such dismissals of HIV as a western demonisation of 'Africa' and the sexuality projected onto it, help explain why in the 1990s, Michael and his friends, who knew the conventional medical story of HIV, 'took it light' and continued, as Michael says, with what they knew was supposed to be 'unsafe' sex, despite positive diagnoses:

> **Michael:** My sister she told me 'this {diagnosis} can't be like that, there's no such thing'. . . . I told my family that I'm HIV they ignore it, which means there's no such thing . . . I just continue with my life doing the ordinary things that I've done like I was just around you know, fooling around, busy with girlfriends you know, and all those, so I was just doing the same things. The point is I didn't condomise because I nearly forgot the point that I'm HIV positive, there's no such thing ok.

HIV's spread in southern Africa has also generated competing explanations. The accepted, evidence-based account cites a combination of factors. In the later part of the twentieth century, HIV may have mutated into more resistant and infective forms. Sexual transmission increased through travel and voluntary and forced migration within and across African countries in situations of labour pressure and armed conflict, and in conditions of poverty and ill-health which themselves derive from earlier histories of slavery and colonialism (Barnett and Whiteside, 2006: 139ff.). Increased urbanisation and modernisation changed the organisation of families and sexual relationships. Untreated, even minor sexually transmitted infections (STIs) increased vulnerability. Growing alcohol and drug use also enhanced vulnerability (Morojele *et al.*, 2006). Some infections may have arisen from needle reuse and transfusion. Condoms' social and personal unacceptability (Bermudez Ribiero de la Cruz, 2004) and association with sex work (Iliffe, 2006: 134); their continuing shortage; lack of HIV education; lack of social power that would make that education effective, particularly for women; and other, strongly competing economic and health priorities, also contributed to the virus's spread. In addition, the long, at first unknown African existence of the virus, itself enabled its extensive spread (Iliffe, 2006).

Women's, particularly younger women's, disproportionate infection rates in South African (MacPhail *et al.*, 2002) and other African contexts are generally explained through the physiological factor of easier transmission during heterosexual intercourse and a range of social factors, including women starting sexual activity younger, having sexual relationships with older men whose longer sexual histories give them more likelihood of infection, and marriage also exposing women to older men with whom they are unlikely to practice safer sex (Clark, 2004). Sexual abuse, domestic violence and women's lack of power to negotiate safer sex also play a part, and contribute to the disproportionate infections of young women. Sexual abuse is indisputably frequent in South Africa (Jewkes and Abrahams, 2002) and may be seen as a normal part of 'love' relationships by some (Outwater *et al.*, 2005). South African research, including our own, frequently finds that women who ask for condoms to be used are accused of infidelity, beaten, verbally abused and losing homes and/or economic support (Morrell *et al.*, 2002).

Women are not just 'victims' in the epidemic, however, but active decision-makers. Some young women express pride in their resourcefulness in obtaining what they need from boyfriends with cars, who serve as the 'Minister for Transport' and boyfriends who help with school fees, 'Ministers for Education' (Morrell *et al.*, 2002; Selikow *et al.*, 2002). Such arrangements may mean having unsafe sex if that is what these 'ministers' want. Others develop strategies to avoid the issues of condoms and HIV status, like Andiswa, one of our interviewees, who went to stay in her sister's house, where she could not have sex with her boyfriend, but where she could still claim his financial support for their child.[8] Women as well as men may offset HIV risk against their desire for children; in South Africa this seems particularly the case in rural areas (Morrell *et al.* 2002). Women may endorse their boyfriends' equations of masculinity with many girlfriends, their dislike of condoms, their elisions of love, trust, health and 'flesh to flesh' or 'skin to skin' sex – all of which are especially dangerous for women – and may also endorse boyfriends' commitment to sex as the best and only free pleasure available (Morrell *et al.*, 2002). The pleasures of sexuality, for women as well as men, are notoriously discounted in many developing-world condom programmes (Gysels *et al.* 2005; Matthews *et al.*, 2006) that focus on 'safe' and ignore 'sex'. This is especially true for younger people, for whom condoms can seem just another one of the older generation's tools for repressing their children's sexualities (Campbell *et al.*, 2005). At the same time many men are ready to reconceptualise masculinity, religiously or politically – as some of our interviewees did – or more specifically, around concepts of maturity, responsibility and fatherhood. Men's groups and education programmes for youth in schools often now try to pursue such reformulations of masculinity. Men are also often ambivalent about their resistance to 'safety'. In South Africa the Lotto slogan 'tata ma chance' ('take my chance'), used by young men to justify their multiple unsafe sex experiences, causes some of them considerable anxiety and conflict (Selikow *et al.*, 2002; see also Baylies and Bujra, 2001, Ouzgane and Morrell, 2005).

Having the power to 'negotiate' condom use is thus a complex issue. It is, too, only part of a broader gendered picture that includes non-HIV-related physical and sexual violence against women, and women's lesser access to education and employment, all of which may lessen their power within sexual relationships. Women who have experienced sexual and physical violence – including those recently arrived in South Africa as forced migrants from conflict zones – may have ongoing difficulties from these experiences that limit their ability to address HIV transmission or being HIV positive.[9] In high unemployment economies, women are especially likely to be forced or induced into unsafe sex work or transactional sex. They have fewer economic options than men (Ndingaye, 2005; Selikow *et al.*, 2002) – though South African men, particularly young men, are also economically and socially marginalised (Burns, 2002). These social exclusions and constraints powerfully affect women's and men's relations with each other. Women's access to HIV services is economically and socially restricted – though men are also widely recognised to underuse these services. Some property and inheritance issues disadvantage women; young women often experience specific versions of social disempowerment. Even more than men, women may experience difficulties in talking not just about condoms but about sex generally, with partners and between generations.[10]

Accounts of HIV's especially high prevalence in southern Africa also cite multiple factors, focusing particularly on men migrating for employment, especially in mining, and being forbidden under apartheid to take their wives and families. Domestic and immigrant migrant workers, it is suggested, developed sexual networks that included partners in urban or mining as well as home, often rural areas – a pattern that also seems now to characterise the Indian epidemic's spread. Sex work in areas with migrant workers rarely involved condoms. High rates of alcohol use among migrant workers promoted unsafe sex. Few clinics were available to provide HIV education or STI treatment. Post-apartheid migration in South Africa has involved more and more women moving for employment or to be near their partners, and people from other African countries, and has been characterised by more contact between migrant workers and local neighbourhoods. HIV rates among miners and migrant workers in South Africa are notably high (Campbell, 2003; Williams *et al.*, 2000); Botswana's epidemic seems similarly related to population mobility, while Angolans' lack of mobility owing to prolonged civil war is thought to explain the country's relatively low (4.6 per cent) HIV prevalence (UNAIDS, 2006).

Other contributing factors in southern Africa may be relatively low rates of male circumcision in southern African countries (Williams *et al.*, 2006); differing HIV strains across the continent; lack of coherent government programmes; and a general lack of discussion of HIV in the region, particularly during the 1990s, allowing young people in particular to view sexual intercourse without condoms as safe. Some researchers have suggested that young people's greater orientation towards individualised consumption also mediates HIV, changing attitudes towards sex, money and consumer goods. This shift might be particularly powerful in countries with a newly strong consumer sector such as South Africa. In South Africa, too – as indeed in the rest of Africa – youth's lack of political engagement is frequently remarked (Gumede, 2005; Selikow *et al.*, 2002), and does not favour involvement with HIV campaigns modelled on traditional community-based lines.

HIV's prevalence may itself feed into the crisis. Our research participants sometimes spoke of HIV as an overwhelming tide that would sweep them and the nation before it. That did not stop them talking positively about their relation to the epidemic at other times, for they reported trying to live healthily and almost always safely with the virus. However, for people who are less in touch with HIV services than were most of our interviewees, the virus's ubiquity, and its coexistence with other everyday economic and health crises, may make it hard to respond to (Ciambrone, 2001; Laubscher, 2003; Selikow *et al.*, 2002).

The standard accounts of African HIV epidemics' development overlap with some implicitly or explicitly racist and sexist geographies of transmission. There are accounts of exotic or abusive sexual practices among Africans, and of 'promiscuity' among young people and 'rampant' STIs. There were concerns, in pre-1994 apartheid South Africa, about HIV and 'interracial' relationships (Mbali, 2005). Attempts continue to identify, if not the Patient Zero of US HIV representations (Shilts, 1988) – the individual alleged to have been responsible for much early transmission – at least a Group Zero – sex workers with high frequencies of unprotected sex, truck drivers having unprotected sex over a wide geographical range – or a Place Zero – in the rainforest, whence sexual transgressiveness and the disease entity spread along the corruption-enabling routes of mobility and modernity (Preston, 1994), 'unnatural' in an African context. There is panic about other African illnesses and epidemics (Squire, 1997). All these mythologies are manifest in popular and some academic discourse on AIDS and Africa. Sometimes, 'culture' stands in for 'race' in familiarly sexualised ways, focusing, for instance, on black South African men's sexual abuse of and violence towards women, especially young women, as if this were a phenomenon specific to HIV or indeed unique to South Africa. There is a similarly racialised focus on 'virgin rape', particularly of very young girls, as a curative practice – an occurrence whose high rates and magical rationale, though they have an enormous media profile, are not supported by detailed research (Jewkes, 2004).[11] Traditions of representing women, particularly sex workers, as vectors and vehicles of disease (Patton, 1993), allied to pathologisations of African subjecthood and sexuality, cast HIV positive African women not as subjects struggling with the problems of the pandemic, but as passive victims, or as uncontrollably sexually transgressive. Female interviewees, in 2001 and 2004, were concerned about telling partners and families because of the associated imputation of their own immorality; some had been abused on this account. As Zoleka, whose husband now ignored her and gave her no money for their children, described:

> **Zoleka**: He said I brought it, he had nothing wrong. I said, 'As I am always indoors, how could I have brought it? At times you come home at 3am and 1am, when I don't even know where you come from.' He said I'm lying, there is no such thing.

Discussing HIV and stigma, several women interviewees suggested that even treatment availability would not remove it for women, because of HIV's connections with disallowed sexuality.

It is hardly surprising that some oppositional explanations, in rejecting mythological accounts of HIV's spread in Africa through sexual transgressiveness and modernity, also erase the multifactorial, evidence-based accounts which these mythologies leech onto. Instead, oppositional accounts blame dirty needles, contaminated transfusions and condoms themselves, signifiers of western regimes' attempts to control African sexuality and populations and of the increasing anti-Christian sexualisation of men's and women's relationships. Condoms are said at times to be deliberately faulty mediators of transmission, or even containers of HIV. Malnutrition and illnesses are said to allow transmission through immunosuppression. Again, these accounts can be persuasive, even though they do not explain the realities of the pandemic within southern Africa.

Most HIV organisations within South Africa and other developing-world countries recognise the racism and discrimination that have given rise to the oppositional accounts, without adopting the accounts themselves. Instead, these organisations endorse the more provisional and cautious orthodoxies summarised above. Our South African interviewees, while advancing some religious metatheories of HIV's inception and prevalence, and some theories based in traditional medicine and spiritual beliefs, did not describe HIV as intentionally spread or an artefact of poverty, but endorsed a broadly scientific, evidence-based account. They emphasised that it was a disease, and human, not animal. Some cited migration as a contributing factor;[12] others talked about the breakdown of social structures during and after apartheid. Interviewees said HIV was 'everyone's' concern. Women often remarked on how they had wrongly thought HIV spread through pro-miscuity, so that their own sexual behaviour rendered them exempt. They cited their sexual conventionality, not to stigmatise other women, but to underline the vulnerability of all.

Nevertheless, both the mythologies and the oppositional accounts of HIV origin and spread can, as Michael described, have strong effects. They can make it difficult to contemplate HIV in yourself, to seek diagnosis and treatment, to speak about it. Oppositional accounts can render HIV unimportant, or a colonising western genocide, in the face of which conventional medicines are worthless or dangerous. Michael pictured himself, his family and neighbourhood making light of HIV in the late 1990s. By 2001, though, his relations all accepted his status, and local people came to him for advice about HIV. Our other interviewees gave medically conventional accounts of their status and lives. They had been diagnosed HIV positive; they sought treatment when they could get it; they ate well, exercised and practised safe sex. Oppositional discourses of ARVs did, however, have some impact. Benjamin, enrolled in an ARV pilot, knew how the drugs worked and how effective they were, and campaigned for them – but had still hesitated to take them, afraid of their rumoured side-effects:

> **Benjamin**: The people are listening each and every kind of a rumour. When there is the medicine now, people are backing up you see. Rumours like, more special like to side-effects, the problem each and every medicine do have a side-effect . . . Like, I was one of them,

I was confused too. But I've been toyi- toyi-ing too much in front of these embassies wanting these medicine. But when I read that which explains AZT what kind of side-effects, Nevirapine what kind of side effects and I say 'No I rather stay like this, I did stay as from 92 to 2001 without these drugs, why I'm using these drugs now? Maybe they gonna make me sick.'

This chapter has so far provided brief versions of the different stories about how HIV got to where it is in South Africa today. The stories I have called 'mythologies' rely for their persuasiveness on their associations with racialised meaning systems. The oppositional accounts I have described are persuasively related to the material realities of a colonial and postcolonial history which is certainly not over (Mbembe, 2001). There is a sense in which they are 'true stories' of some aspects of the pandemic. However, the stories I have favoured fit a wider range of HIV's material realities, including those of HIV science. They are flexible enough to address the historical realities of the oppositional stories alongside social, epidemiological and physiological realities. This is indeed how many of our research participants treated them, as accounts that could be drawn on pragmatically to make sense of the epidemic, in conjunction with other religious and personal accounts.

The next section of this chapter presents a brief history of South African responses to the epidemic, in which the stories described above interact with national political, social and economic realities.[13]

The HIV epidemic in South Africa

In South Africa in 1990, HIV prevalence among pregnant women was 0.76 per cent; by 2000 it was 22.4 per cent (Abdool Karim and Abdool Karim, 2002). Deaths in 2005 were estimated at 320,000 – around 0.8 per cent of the population (Statistics South Africa, 2001; UNAIDS, 2006). These are inexact measures of the epidemic's development, but they give a sense of its expansion and scope.

The first recorded AIDS deaths in South Africa were in 1982, among white gay men. There were certainly cases in the heterosexual population during the 1980s – somewhat later than in East and Central Africa (Lutambi, 2005). But at this time, HIV was seen largely as a disease of westerners, white gay men and drug users – non-African, sexually transgressive 'others' (Joffe, 1997), though sometimes 'other' Africans were also thought responsible. AIDS deaths also tended, as in the early stages of other countries' epidemics, to be attributed to something 'other', such as TB, malaria or hunger.

During apartheid, the ANC was at the forefront of demanding action on AIDS. Lesbian and gay activists working within the anti-apartheid struggle were key HIV campaigners.[14] In 1992, Mandela helped form the National AIDS Convention of South Africa; the two first post-apartheid health ministers, Dr Nkososana Zuma and Dr Manto Tshabalala-Msimang, were both members.[15] By now, heterosexual cases had overtaken those among homosexual men. In 1994, the year of the first democratic elections, South Africa's first community-based HIV organisation, the National Association of People Living with AIDS (NAPWA), formed to fight discrimination and stigmatisation. HIV was addressed through the post-apartheid government's Reconstruction and Development Programme, or RDP, which pledged to provide good health care for everyone; the health budget rose for several years and facilities were desegregated. However, HIV was not a major priority, something Mandela later acknowledged as a mistake. Top of the RDP agenda came employment, land, houses, services such as water and electricity, education and general health.

South Africa's controversial, World Bank-influenced structural adjustment programme, the Growth Employment and Redistribution Strategy, or GEAR, began in 1996. This effort to make South Africa a globally competitive economy superceded the RDP, under which the rand had weakened and the economy looked unstable. Now, public–private partnerships, labour flexibility, trade liberalisation and sound fiscal policy became – as had happened in the developed world over the past 15 years – key. GEAR seemed to many to depart from the pledges of the Constitution and to ignore the government's mandate to help the poor and underprivileged. In the late 1990s, despite a balanced budget and a strengthening rand, there were job losses in manufacturing and other sectors (except retail and finance), no compensating rise in external or internal investment, and a drop in social spending, including on health.[16] As in other developing-world contexts, structural adjustment worsened health (Farmer, 1999). In 1996, nevertheless, the South African government spent highly on one HIV project: R14m went to *Sarafina 2*, a musical about the schoolgirl anti-apartheid activist of the first 1988 *Sarafina* production, now presented as an HIV social worker. To public disquiet, this lavishly funded production played in a few places, sending out a partial prevention message mainly about condoms, and making no reference to relationships, gender or even the main tenet of the then-dominant ABC strategy, abstention.[17]

A major shift towards public acceptance of HIV in South Africa happened with the death of Gugu Dlamini. In late 1998, this Durban NAPWA activist was beaten to death by a group of local people, including some of her neighbours, shortly after disclosing, on World AIDS Day, that she was HIV positive. This murder was nationally and internationally decried; three years later, many of our interviewees remembered and mentioned it. Thabo Mbeki himself said, 'It is a terrible story. We have to treat people who have HIV with care and support, and not as if they have an illness that is evil'.[18]

Just before Dlamini's murder, Simon Nkoli, a prominent HIV activist who had a long history of anti-apartheid and gay and lesbian activism, and was one of the first openly gay members of the ANC, had died of AIDS. These two events were followed by the establishment at the end of 1998 of the Treatment Action Campaign. TAC, probably the most effective HIV organisation in South Africa, was formed by a group including Zackie

Achmat, another long-term anti-apartheid and lesbian and gay rights activist and longtime ANC member, and other HIV activists. From the start, TAC connected HIV to issues such as TB, malaria, general ill-health, poverty, crime and gender violence. However, it focused on the increasing need for ARVs, now dramatically reducing AIDS deaths in the developed world, for the growing numbers ill enough, like Nkoli, to require treatment. It moved HIV activism in South Africa from its early emphasis on confidentiality to stressing openness, and then treatment.

ARVs seemed to many developed-world funders and NGOs to be prohibitively expensive and complex for the developing world, requiring sophisticated and unending treatment regimes, and extra infrastructure, medical capacity and training. In addition, some in the South African government saw ARVs as toxic and colonising. However, they were clearly potentially affordable and feasible for stopping mother-to-child HIV transmission, for which only brief treatment was required, and it was this project that first occupied TAC.[19]

TAC has shown, as organisations such as ACT UP in the US, the Terrence Higgins Trust in the UK and TASO in Uganda did in the early days of their epidemics, the effectiveness that civil society organisations can have, particularly those driven largely by people who are HIV affected and infected. TAC works with local neighbourhoods, similar organisations nationally and transnationally, and international supporters, globalising 'from below' (Brecher *et al.*, 2000; Robins, 2004) but retaining a locally and nationally 'rooted cosmopolitanism' (Tarrow, 2005: 42). It mobilises politically on issues that the state and political parties are neglecting, to create powerful alliances around those issues – in TAC's case, with the AIDS Law Project, Médecins sans Frontières (MSF), the South African Medical Association, and the Congress of South African Trades Unions (COSATU) and the South African Communist Party – the two political partners of the main government party, the African National Congress or ANC. Many TAC members are in the ANC and it has also consistently tried to work with government. It expertly cultivates the media, and has worked with them to change the terms of public debate. It employs diverse actions, symbolic as well as practical, that include all its members – court cases, lobbying, letters to newspapers, media campaigns, posters and fliers, petitions, street demonstrations, singing and die-ins, and HIV Positive T-shirts for all to wear, irrespective of status, drawing everyone into the HIV political community – Nelson Mandela himself was pictured wearing one. The organisation draws on traditions of anti-apartheid struggle from the 1950s through to the 1980s, but also those of the gay and lesbian movement in South Africa, and of HIV activism globally, in particular the media-aware and popular culture-orientated strategies of ACT UP (Crimp and Ralston, 1990; Mbali, 2005). It includes a wide range of members: a large number of unemployed and poor black activists, mainly women; people of all ethnicities with histories of anti-apartheid activism; younger working-class black people; middle-class professionals, mainly white. TAC's treatment campaigns, unlike those developed by HIV activists in the US, were tied from the start to broader political analyses. At the same time, many of its analyses and goals were close to those of international organisations such as MSF, WHO and UNAIDS, which some in the South Africa, like other developing-world countries, see as having incipiently neo-colonial agendas.

TAC's first actions occurred at a time of increasing representations of HIV in the media and in public health campaigns. In 1999, Thabo Mbeki replaced Mandela as President and began the loveLife HIV awareness campaign, organised by a coalition of NGOs and funded both governmentally and privately, predominantly by the Department of Health and the Kaiser Foundation.[20] loveLife aims at getting adolescents to make informed life choices around health, sexuality and education, but also targets parents, educators and concerned older adults. Its initial tag line, 'talk about it', was followed in later years by the aspirational 'love to be there', the self-affirmational 'get attitude', and most recently and confrontationally, 'HIV-Face It'. The campaign involves youth work as well as public education; loveLife sponsors around 1500 groundBREAKER peer educators a year, many of whom acquire skills meant to enhance their employment chances. However, it is best known for its billboards showing young racially diverse but mostly black people, often in girl-boy pairs, in settings related to relationships and sexuality, education and careers. Previous loveLife campaigns received a great deal of criticism for an inexplictness – talk about what? And then, do what? – that often left audiences confused, as with similar campaigns in, for instance, the 1980s in the early days of the UK epidemic which showed icebergs and tombstones against the cryptic slogan, 'AIDS – don't die of ignorance'. loveLife has also been criticised for the apparent affluence of the billboard models – when HIV affects a largely poor population; the urban, English (although urban South Africans mostly speak some English), western-inflected language of the campaigns; its emphasis on sex, particularly heterosexual intercourse;[21] its youth-oriented discourse and activities, promoting peer at the expense of family relationships; and its brand and consumer-focused approach. These criticisms highlight the many dimensions traversing the global/local nexus of HIV awareness campaigns, reminding us that the 'cultures' engaged by such billboards are never stable or unified but always shifting, being 'cultivated' (Mercer, 1994; Mkhise, 2004). loveLife is also questioned over its contradictory presentation of sex as both natural and requiring expert talk, and for its assumption, ignoring considerations of gendered and generational power, that such talk is a catch-all solution (Wilbraham, 2004). However, awareness and approval of the programmes among young people is high (Reproductive Health Research Unit/loveLife, 2004). Perhaps some talk about sexualities and 'the big thing', however confused, has been better than none at all. loveLife has tried to work in the gap between stigmatised, silenced sexualities, and sex talk as itself a coercive, colonising imperative (Foucault, 1979; Heath, 1982). Its most recent campaigns, while still high on production values, engage with HIV, condoms and gender inequities with considerable directness.[22]

A contrasting media programme had begun in 1994. The *Soul City* 'edutainment' foundation produced a TV and radio drama with spin-off projects such as magazines and advocacy groups. Centred on a clinic, each series addressed HIV alongside other health issues such as infant health and asthma, as well as more general concerns such as violence against women, xenophobia and volunteering. The 2003 television series was watched at some time by 65 per cent of adults and nearly half of these reported watching 'most' episodes. A similar set of series for children around 8 to 12, *Soul Buddyz*, also runs. Building on a 50-year history of health edutainment for social change in Africa, *Soul City* has become a continent-wide – and indeed worldwide exemplar of broadcast HIV education, and of crossregional and transnational media processes at work outside the 'developed' world. Exposure to *Soul City* radio, television and print materials is not always easy to disentangle from other factors in people's lives, but it seems to correlate with helpful changes in HIV and other attitudes.[23] In 2001, *Soul City* was often the only place people heard HIV talked about in an accepting and affirmative way. For some interviewees, the programmes constituted their first, virtual HIV support 'community'.

The media's increasing openness in the approach to the new millennium, was also mirrored in public figures. There was little mention of HIV/AIDS during the 1999 election campaign (Uys, 2003: 113). But in the same year, Graça Machel, widow of Mozambique's deceased president, and wife of Nelson Mandela, placed a death notice for her brother-in-law, Boaventura Moises Machel, declaring AIDS the cause of death. This frankness was widely noted both in Mozambique and in South Africa where – as in other HIV epidemics – obituarial silence or euphemisms, such as 'TB' and 'a long illness', still dominate. In the same year, Judge Edwin Cameron, a well-known figure of legal resistance to apartheid, declared himself HIV positive and used his own case as evidence that antiretroviral drugs worked.[24]

Despite this increased level of representation, treatment initiatives were not progressing. While a few HIV positive people had access to ARVs through research trials or private clinics, the government refused to provide them, and suspended doctors who prescribed them, even if only to prevent sero-conversion after sexual assault. It wanted to find an African alternative to neo-colonial dependency for life, and a lifetime, on multinational pharmaceutical corporations. However, the main South African candidate, 'Virodene', containing a substance previously used as an industrial solvent and developed by a Pretoria pharmaceutical company, was concluded in 1999 to be toxic and without effects on HIV disease.[25] In 2000, the government voiced the possibility that ARVs were useless remedies being imposed on Africa in economically ruinous and potentially racist ways. President Mbeki began investigating the work of mainly US AIDS 'denialists' such as David Rasnick and Peter Duesberg who claimed that HIV was a harmless virus; that 'AIDS' resulted from other health and nutrition problems, from ARVs themselves or – for western gay men – overuse of recreational drugs; that HIV was not a serious issue in South Africa; and that most 'AIDS' deaths were in fact due to other illnesses, and to the main underlying cause: poverty.[26]

Similar arguments had achieved currency in the developed world when AZT, a toxic and difficult to tolerate anti-cancer drug, was the only available ARV treatment. In US support groups I worked with as a volunteer in the late 1980s and early 1990s, people often found AZT making them iller than HIV and so stopped taking it and started using alternative treatments. For a short while, their health might improve; invariably, it later failed. By 2000, effective and much less toxic ARV regimes were in place in the developed world; AIDS denialists had much less purchase there. They started to address their arguments to the developing world, where ARVs were rarely available or affordable. Some also sold their own very expensive remedies. In July 2000, Mbeki invited both orthodox and dissident HIV scientists to form a presidential advisory panel. The resultant report exhibited a stalemate disagreement on the cause of AIDS and the nature of HIV.[27]

The government argued that ARVs, even in cheap, short-term MTCT programmes, were dangerous as they had not been fully tested in the African context. The toxicity argument had been raised vociferously against MTCT in its earliest US days by a women's group within ACT UP. Trials later demonstrated the treatment's safety, and it was endorsed even before that by the women recruited to trials, whose priority was to have healthy children. Women within TAC were expressing this same powerful priority. A South African study showed, moreover, that MTCT would be considerably cheaper than treating HIV positive children (Skordis and Nattrass, 2001). Another, less explicit government concern was the long-term cost of HIV positive women having HIV negative children whom the state would later have to support.[28]

In 2000 at the International AIDS Conference in Durban, Mbeki's keynote speech emphasised poverty's role in HIV/AIDS. Also at this conference, Nkosi Johnson, then 11 years old, became the first black South African to speak publicly to a wide audience about living with AIDS, broadcasting a plea for knowledge and acceptance, an extract from which begins this chapter: 'You can't get AIDS if you touch, hug, kiss, hold hands with someone who is infected . . . don't be afraid of us – we are all the same.' This event received extensive media attention nationwide, and internationally. Johnson himself emphasised the need for pregnant HIV positive women to receive publicly-funded MTCT treatment; Mbeki left the conference during the speech. Mandela's (2000) closing speech at the conference called for action against HIV,[29] 'one of the greatest threats humankind has faced', and – again – for antiretroviral treatment for HIV positive pregnant women. Mandela is of course no ordinary ex-president, but one still held in extremely high regard. While he repeatedly emphasised his support for Mbeki on AIDS as on other issues, our research participants often contrasted his position with that of Mbeki, and speculated about a happier prognosis for the epidemic had he not stepped down.

Aside from Mandela, there was considerable internal dissent in the governing ANC. The committee on Joint Monitoring Committee on the Improvement of the Quality of Life and Status of Women supported MTCT and ARV treatment for sexual assault victims. Its chair, Pregs Govender, accused the ANC of moving from collectivism to 'groupthink'. However, the firm structures of the party, and its history as a democratic-centralist organisation when banned and in exile – arguably contributing to its later defensiveness over external and internal, political and civil society criticism (Govender, 2006; Hemson and O'Donovan, 2006) – all made changing its approach to HIV difficult. Moreover, the ANC's emerging future as an organisation driven less by mass involvement than by expertise, something along the lines of the UK's New Labour, concerns about internal destabl- isation so soon into democracy and ANC MPs' worries about the career effects of going off-message, did not encourage explicit disagreement (Gumede, 2005). The South African scientific establishment, though, was unambiguous in its condemnation. The then-President of the Medical Research Council, Malegapuru William Makgoba, editor of *African Renais- sance* (1999), to which Mbeki wrote the Prologue, dismissed AIDS dissidence as 'pseudoscience' and pointed out its unAfrican origins (2000).

Next year, during our research interviews, Johnson, although by then taking ARVs provided by a benefactor, became very sick. He asked to see Mbeki. Mbeki's wife, Zanele, visited instead. Johnson died in June. Many of our research participants mentioned both his landmark HIV-disclosing speech, and the government's lack of respect for him. 'He should have gone himself, not sent his wife', Yoliswa commented. Not just the absence of treatment provision, but also this political distancing, along with a sense that the government was not interested in the poor, created a gap between the government – Mbeki in particular – and a group that was now an important part of its political constituency: people living with HIV.[30]

Like the government, TAC criticised the power of western drug com- panies, and explicitly compared resistance to them to the mass civil disobedience of the 1950s, the Defiance Campaign against apartheid Pass Laws. Between 2000 and 2001 it operated a successful Defiance Campaign of its own to get generic fluconazole, an effective treatment for HIV-related cryptococcal meningitis and thrush, available in public health facilities, after one of its activists, Christopher Moraka – after whom the campaign was named – died, while suffering from systemic thrush.[31] Trying to get Pfizer, who sold a patented version in South Africa, to reduce its prices to generic level or relax its patent, TAC illegally imported and distributed stocks of a generic equivalent drug from Thailand, and pushed through an obstacle course of medical bureaucracy and government legal uncertainty to get the generic's import and distribution licensed (Achmat, 2001). This process was still happening during our research. Interviewees in some places had good access to fluconazole; in others it was rarely available. However, its recent arrival was generally viewed as a hopeful sign of HIV treatment advance, presaging the coming of ARVs. For the few research participants who had participated in the fluconazole Defiance Campaign demonstrations, this was a powerful personal and collective victory, legitimised in the courts but achieved by their own actions.[32]

Later in 2001, the government was sure enough of its legal ground to defeat, with TAC as a 'friend of the court', a case brought by international pharmaceutical companies that challenged South Africa's right to import and manufacture cheap, generic drugs. That same year, though, TAC itself brought a case against the government, claiming that MTCT rollout to the whole country, and ARV treatment for people who had been sexually assaulted, were state obligations. The case was accompanied by multiple local meetings, marches and other actions, including a poster campaign that featured an image of the recently deceased Nkosi Johnson alongside the famous 1976 picture of Hector Pieterson, the 13-year-old killed by the police during the 1976 Soweto student uprising. This visual paralleling of apartheid and democratic postapartheid governments 'killing' children caused controversy, even among those who rejected the government's line on ARVs. However, the parallel was also made by Bishop Desmond Tutu, who called for a struggle against the epidemic to match the struggle against apartheid.

In response to the TAC campaign, government members began a long-running trend of accusing TAC of being run by whites and in the pay of pharmaceutical companies. TAC, however, has continued to pursue collaboration with the ANC and the government wherever feasible, on the shared constitutional health principles of Batho Pele – People First.

TAC won the 2001 case, but the government appealed, resulting in a year delay.[33] Rollout of treatment for pregnant HIV positive women still took a long time and is not yet complete. Some provinces acted early, particularly the Western Cape which initiated a programme in 2001 for its relatively small numbers of HIV positive pregnant women. This was facilitated by its provincial government being controlled by the Democratic Alliance, therefore not tied to the ANC-dominated government line on antiretrovirals, and having particularly strong periurban health service infrastructure and management (Naimak, 2006). Many of our women interviewees had experienced the Western Cape programme, entering it after voluntary HIV counselling and testing (VCT) during antenatal care. The programme found over 90 per cent of babies tested at nine months HIV negative (Abdullah *et al.*, 2002), even though, unlike in most developed world programmes, some mothers were very ill with AIDS, and some breast-fed. Followup testing has been difficult, typically covering around 50 per cent of infants, due to population mobility and lack of transport (Jones *et al.*, 2005). Recent studies also suggest that breast-feeding remains the best option for the many HIV-positive women – including some in rural South Africa – who do not have access to clean water (World Health Organisation, 2006b).

Among research participants whose babies had been tested, all were negative, and the scheme had had major educative and health benefits for the women themselves. Interviewees who had experience of MTCT programmes spontaneously said very good things about their government's approach to HIV issues, asking only that ARV treatment now be extended to them as well as their babies.

In July 2003, Mbeki declared he knew no one who had died of HIV (*Washington Post*, 30 July 2003), despite persistent rumours that two of his close political colleagues who opposed ARVs had died of AIDS. Media portrayed Mbeki as in his own world, a view shared by many of our iller interviewees, who wondered whether wealth or political privilege were shielding government members from knowledge of their poorer constituents' sufferings. Certainly, MPs can always access ARVs themselves, through the private health care schemes to which they are subscribed.

In the continuing absence of a treatment plan, TAC brought a charge of culpable homicide against the health and trade ministers, using 'wanted for homicide' posters strongly reminiscent of those flyposted by ACT UP against US President Reagan. It also instituted a civil disobedience campaign much criticised by the government, calling for a national treatment plan. TAC's Zackie Achmat refused to take ARVs until they were available to all, despite his own severe HIV-illnesses. Acceding to activists' requests, Achmat started treatment in August 2003, shortly afterwards the government unveiled its Comprehensive HIV/AIDS Care, Management and Treatment Plan, and TAC called off its civil disobedience campaign.

Treatment rollout for people who meet WHO criteria for antiretroviral therapy is still being critically assessed against its implementation. By the end of 2005 190,000 were thought to be provided for, around 20 per cent of those who needed it (UNAIDS, 2006). This failure to meet the 50 per cent specifications in the UN '3 by 5' plan can be attributed to high demand, the drain of trained staff to high-income countries, medical supply problems and, allegedly, government reluctance and its local manifestations in some provinces' slow compliance with the treatment plan. Treatment rollout delays were, for instance, powerfully protested against in early 2005 by TAC activists in the Eastern Cape, 40 of whom were injured by rubber bullets and smoke grenades fired by the police (Mtathi, 2005).

Pilot studies of ARVs suggested good adherence and 80 per cent survival after 18 months (Orrell *et al.*, 2003; Médecins sans Frontières and World Health Organisation, 2003).[34] The health minister, Manto Tshabalala-Msimang, however, raised concerns about people dying on ARVs, or leaving treatment, and appeared to view the treatment figures as worryingly large, rather than small. She resisted answering to WHO-set targets, apparently seeing this organisation, as do many, developing-world politicians, as non-consultative and Eurocentric; and she repeatedly set against ARVs the role of good nutrition in combating HIV.

A picture of treatment provision for our South African interviewees in townships near Cape Town gives some indication of the difficulties and changes. In 2001, the Western Cape was something of a treatment exception in South Africa. Not just voluntary VCT, but MTCT, were available to all in the province. Some medications for opportunistic infections were provided in public clinics; as interviewees reported though, they often ran out, were much too expensive for them to buy in the private sector, and corporate employers' provision of them was much lower than their public declarations suggested. The primary ARV provision in reality was through a charity programme for children, which had been available for some years, and a small NGO pilot. A hospital also ran ARV trials in which, on compassionate grounds, medications were continued to participants almost indefinitely, though flexibility of prescription was limited. All of these were used by some interviewees. Hospital, clinic and private doctors and nurses referred patients to the latter two programmes whenever possible; several interviewees were waiting for such referrals to be taken up.

The Western Cape began general ARV treatment earlier than the rest of South Africa, often delivering to the now-treatment-literate women who had been in its MTCT programmes, mobilising NGOs and CBOs involved with those programmes and getting early support from the Global Fund to fight AIDS, Tuberculosis and Malaria. By 2003–4, all research participants who needed ARVs could access them, through a mixture of national, provincial, NGO (MSF) and Global Fund programmes. At first, the rollout was slow and understaffed – a hospital's HIV clinic might only have one doctor working at a time, who could also have other hospital responsibilities. The programme also required patients to make pre-treatment visits over, usually, four weeks. Patients with TB had to engage successfully in TB treatment for two months if not previously treated.[35] These were difficult conditions when 60 per cent of people with TB in the area were also HIV positive, and when people waiting for treatment were seriously ill. When we tried to recontact our 2001 research participants in 2003, two were reported to have died while waiting for ARV treatment to start, or during its early days.[36] Four of the eight we recontacted were doing well on ARVs, reflecting findings in larger studies of ARVs and 'quality of life' in this neighbourhood (Jelsma *et al.*, 2005). Most of our other 24 HIV-positive interviewees had been diagnosed while still well. Some, according to CBO and NGO workers, had moved, and most others were reported to be well. This apparently large proportion of continuing healthy 2001 interviewees testifies to the effectiveness of the province's encouragement, through VCT and MTCT programmes, of early testing. Khayelitsha, the large township that was local to many of our interviewees, has an HIV test rate of 41 per cent (Ndingaye, 2005). In 2006, the Western Cape provided ARVs for around 8,000 people – perhaps 65 per cent of those needing them, at 45 sites (Naimak, 2006; Overseas Development Institute, 2006). On World AIDS Day 2006, it even launched a comprehensive 'Get Tested' campaign providing drop-in HIV testing services in shopping malls as well as clinics, drawing on Washington DC's similar initiative earlier in the year.

There continues to be government disquiet over racialised modes of explaining HIV, which tends to work against prioritising HIV treatment. In 2004, for instance, President Mbeki wrote in the weekly online journal *ANC Today* about racism's continuing legacy, addressing some critical accounts of South Africa's sexual crime statistics. Mbeki wanted to oppose the slippage from concern about sexual crime, to whites' irrational pathologisation of black men. 'For (whites)', he wrote, 'our new democracy feels fraught with threats ... fear of crime becomes the concentrated expression of fear about their survival in a sea of black savages' (Mbeki, 2004a, b). This article was referred to shortly afterwards in a parliamentary question from opposition Democratic Alliance MP Ryan Coetzee about links between sexual violence and HIV. Responding, Mbeki refused to address HIV; this indeed is the speech from which his words at the start of this chapter come. Instead, he expanded his consideration of racialisation, citing writers from South Africa and elsewhere as ANC theorists have done on this topic throughout the party's history. This parliamentary reply was extensively quoted by the media in South Africa and abroad, usually with no distinction drawn between Mbeki's and others' words. In particular there was dismay at the use of the words below – phrases that come, as Mbeki indicated, from an article by the African–American professor, Edward Rymes:

> People ... have written that our cultures, religion and social norms as Africans condition us to be 'rampant sexual beasts, unable to control our urges, unable to keep our legs crossed, unable to keep it in our pants' – the rapists the Hon Coetzee says that, 'in large part ... (account) for the spread of HIV in the country.'
>
> (Mbeki, 2004b)

For Mbeki, HIV discourse – like the abuse discourse – is, then, often a sexualising racism. But this was not the economic and political language in which racism is usually discussed by the South African Parliament, the ANC or Mbeki himself, which may partly explain the shocked reactions to it.[37] It was literally not Mbeki's language either, though he was understood as endorsing it.

Mbeki's frustration with what he views as racist pathologisations of Africa is comprehensible, especially given South Africa's focus on the African Renaissance (Makgoba, 1999), in which African 'culture' and 'tradition' play important and ideal, even idealised, roles. Women's place within this renaissance is however an ambiguous one (Msimang, 2000). Mbeki's words can also be read as a refusal to take sexual violence seriously, and as a further example of the government's widely cited 'AIDS denialism'.[38]

Despite these political ambiguities, the trend towards more openness about HIV continued, especially among public figures. When in 2001 we began the research interviews, the media and everyday conversations were already saturated with references to HIV. Though disclosure of one's own status was rare, family members were increasingly mentioned as affected. In 2003, Fana Khaba – the DJ who later switched from ARVs to Africa's Solution – declared his HIV positive status, gaining massive support. In 2004, Mangosuthu Buthelezi, leader of the opposition Inkatha Freedom Party, spoke at his son's funeral of AIDS as the cause of death. Mandela openly discussed the death of his eldest son from AIDS in early 2005. After the 2004 implementation of the national plan, Mbeki spoke a little more on the topic. In his 2005 State of the Nation address he declared that this plan, 'among the best in the world, combining awareness, treatment and home-based care, is being implemented with greater vigour' (Mbeki, 2005; see also Department of Health, 2005b). The government also supported, from 2002 to 2006, a post-ABC, post-loveLife education and awareness campaign, Khomanani, 'Caring together for life', in collaboration with the *Soul City* trust and private sector companies. Its aims – 'to Care; to Talk; to Test; to Condomise' – went along with six priorities: orphans and young children, youth, health workers, healthy positive living, treating STIs and treating TB. Khomanani was explicit about safety, addressed treatment and evaluated its programmes in ways not previously associated with government HIV campaigns. However, government continues to grant HIV a dangerously low priority, given its significance in people's lives. Internationally it is seen, as Stephen Lewis, UN special envoy on AIDS, phrased it, as 'obtuse, dilatory and negligent' about treatment rollout (*New York Times*, 7 September 2006).

One index of political lack of commitment to a serious, scientifically and socially founded approach to HIV is the long-running case of Mathias Rath. In mid-2005, another putative African Solution appeared when Rath, a US businessman with an internet vitamin company claiming to cure cancer and AIDS, started visiting townships around Cape Town. He distributed vitamins, some of them possibly dangerous for people with poor immune functioning, conducted an unauthorised 'trial' of their effectiveness, and gave out fliers claiming that: ARVs were poisonous; AIDS could be cured with proper nutrition, including his vitamins; and TAC, the UN and World Bank, UK Chancellor Gordon Brown and US President George Bush were all in the pay of multinational pharmaceutical companies. Rath also ran full-page advertisements in US and South African newspapers urging donors to achieve 'health for all by the Year 2020' (*New York Times*, 6 May 2005). Rath's advertisements have been banned by a number of national advertising authorities and his activities condemned by WHO, UNAIDS and UNICEF. TAC successfully applied to the courts to stop his accusations against it, and he has been criticised by senior ANC MPs. He has won some support from traditional healers – though many others prefer to collaborate with western medicine around HIV. However, his apparent Afrocentrism and emphasis on nutrition appealed to some government members. The health minister, facetiously known as Dr Garlic, suggested his operations were a free speech issue, praised nutritional addresses to HIV, and at the same time remarked, with ill-advised flippancy, on the helpfulness of garlic and lemon juice for the complexion as well as the immune system (*Guardian*, 6 May 2005). Multivitamins are relatively widely available, free, in public clinics, for people with HIV. Yet in some cases, people who are medical candidates for ARVs, as well as others already being treated, reportedly adopted Rath's programme, sometimes with very negative results (Treatment Action Campaign, 2005).

Nutrition is agreed to be crucial in managing HIV disease, though conventional medical approaches emphasise it cannot function in place of ARVs (Fawzi *et al.*, 2004). The Rath phenomenon and similar events, like the positive responses to Tina van der Maas's nutritional regime, are partly indicators of continuing shortages of ARV treatment, and ARV education, in South Africa. In addition, they are indicators of a second, 'post-treatment' epidemic. In this second epidemic, people are living, like HIV positive people in the developed world, with ARV use and its problems. This second epidemic is characterised by short-term and long-term side-effects of some ARVs such as rashes; lipodystrophy, which can create wasting of the face and legs and thickening around the waist; neuropathy, usually manifesting as severe pain in the feet and legs; and growing resistance to or failures in efficacy of some medications. In addition – unlike in the developed world – problems with first- and second-line ARVs are, given patent restrictions and government inaction on accessing alternatives, proving hard to solve. As in the early days of developed-world ARV treatment, support is even less available for such issues than it is for ARV treatment itself. Side-effects' physiological and psychological significance are often ignored unless judged medically significant. Economic hardships may increase: ARVs make you healthier, hungrier and remove your entitlement to disability grant. If you are unemployed, travel to clinics and buying enough food becomes even harder. As with other serious chronic illnesses, you may live in an uncertain state, by turns 'healthy' and 'sick'. Forms of treatment, support and activism developed for the earlier phases of the epidemic have, as in other countries, to shift in order to address these new difficulties in people's relations with the virus. This is, then, a developing-world version of the time 'after' HIV crisis, the time of HIV as a treatable condition, featuring some of the same issues faced since the late 1990s in developed-world HIV epidemics. But it is occuring alongside the 'first' epidemic of untreated HIV and is thus more a continuance of crisis than a post-crisis state. Moreover, given the unaddressed difficulties of this 'second epidemic', a vitamin cure may sound a distinct improvement upon lifelong medication with side-effects.

The 'second epidemic' is also characterised by the new generation of young people, South Africa's 'born-frees', becoming HIV vulnerable: people who do not remember a time before free condoms and loveLife billboards. It may involve overburdening, as it has in other high HIV-prevalence contexts (Gilbert and Wright, 2002), when increasing numbers of friends and family die, and more people become ill and dependent on those who are still well. 'HIV fatigue' may set in, even among those infected, particularly when research and resources all seem to be directed at HIV. To many, it now seems invidious to privilege those who are HIV positive but well, over those who are HIV negative but poorer or sicker.

Contemporary government discourse is trying to address the ubiquity and the shifting state of HIV. It acknowledges HIV as a problem for everyone. People in South Africa are all 'living with HIV', and the virus is no longer presented only as an adjunct to generalised poverty and ill health. HIV education and social programmes are directed at whole neighbourhoods, rather than simply at the HIV positive – and this seems an effort to be inclusive about HIV, rather than deny it. Government also addresses at least some gendered aspects of the epidemic. For instance, it has declared virginity testing as an HIV preventative as unconstitutional. The strategy is widely decried by women's organisations also for being ineffective, sexually stigmatising women, liable to encourage violence and adopting a view of 'African' culture as singular, static and fixed in the past.[39]

At the same time, Rath's successes and similar phenomena occur within South Africa's continuing history of government ambivalence about HIV transmission and treatment, linked to its resistance to international organisations' neo-colonial development and health initiatives. In these circumstances, it is unsurprising that considerable contradictions emerge. In 2006, the trial and acquittal of former Vice-President Jacob Zuma on charges of raping an HIV positive woman, raised again the relation of AIDS denialism to gender relations and gender violence. Zuma's previous involvement with HIV issues had seemed relatively informed. A candidate to succeed Mbeki as ANC leader, he has also been associated with a 'pro-poor' economic agenda. In court, he justified what he described as unprotected consensual intercourse with the woman on the grounds that men were less at risk, and that he had showered afterwards. The HIV sector expressed comprehensive dismay (*Mail* and *Guardian*, 8 April 2006). TAC asked Zuma to apologise and engage in HIV education with communities he represents, and while eschewing political positions, called for a future ANC leader who was both committed to HIV issues and pro-poor in their policies. One positive step was that Zuma's successor, Phumzile Mlambo-Ngcuka, committed herself to an integrated attempt to 'defeat this disease' through ARV-based treatment and increased prevention and education (*Guardian*, 28 October 2006), and began developing a new National Strategic Plan to address HIV in South Africa up to 2011, now (March 2007) in a draft consultative form (Department of Health, 2007). The plan is being coordinated by an acting health minister, Jeff Radebe, as Tshabalala-Msimang herself has health problems.

The government has, since 2005, been more explicitly committed to poverty reduction and opposed to the rampant consumerism Mbeki decries. In 2006 it produced a report, *A Nation in the Making*, emphasising the need to build 'social capital' and social cohesion.[40] It briefly mentions HIV mortality as contributing to this need, but gives little space to the epidemic. Moreover, despite maintaining a safe distance from World Bank loans and building alliances with progressive governments in Africa and across the developing world, the government still endorses a market-led economy. It has, for instance, proposed a shift to social health insurance, whose burden would fall largely on the working poor, including those with HIV. With 50 per cent living in poverty and almost that number unemployed, there are increasing levels of protest over rent and utility charges ramped up by newly privatised corporations. Government is frequently perceived as building the black bourgeoisie, promoting 'Black Economic Empowerment' for the few, at the expense of 'a better life for all'. The tripartite alliance between the ANC, COSATU and the South African Communist Party has weakened; calls for a new opposition party are frequent. A recent expression of opposition was the People's Budget cowritten by COSATU, the South Africa coalition of NGOs, and the South African Council of Churches. This document strongly supports a Basic Income Grant form of social security, a campaign that TAC and many other civil society organisations endorse, and opposes the new health plans as a move away from public health as guaranteed in the Constitution (COSATU, 2005; see also Freund, 2006; Gumede, 2005; Hart, 2002; Kingsnorth, 2003; Naidoo and Veriava, 2003).

At the level of neighbourhoods, to which policy concerns with social capital are now tending, working against HIV continues to involve local specificity and alliances. A pragmatic building-up of concepts and actions remains a more appropriate response than a rush to assume overarching theoretical and practical commonalities. Such pragmatism produces ways of thinking and acting that, while they do not look like elite 'theory' (West, 1989: 231), themselves constitute the effective 'theory' of the epidemic. This is something that has happened elsewhere in the pandemic, for instance, in Haiti, where Farmer (1999) describes successful projects as governed by 'pragmatic solidarity',[41] and India, where workers may reflect on the practical conditions of their lives and their wider gendered and employment context in ways that sometimes allow – though they sometimes inhibit – effective action to reduce HIV transmission (Cornish, 2004). This pragmatism is also apparent in some of the advice-orientated texts written about the South African epidemic (for instance, Mahlangu-Ngcobo, 2001).

A practical example of such a response in South Africa occurred in the wake of the death, in December 2003, in Khayelitsha, of Lorna Mlofana, a TAC HIV treatment literacy educator, who was raped by several young men. After she told them she was HIV positive they beat her to death. At such times, it might seem that responses to the epidemic have not progressed since Gugu Dlamini's murder. However, this incident was reported in the press as an untypical criminal act, signalling how far things had come since that murder. Local attitudes were said by Mlofana's colleagues (Naimak, 2006) to be very different now, broadly supportive of people living with HIV. The crime led to a neighbourhood campaign lasting throughout the investigation, trial and eventual conviction two years later of Mlofana's murderer. This campaign, involving TAC and other CBOs, pursued justice for Mlofana, but also argued for better rape crisis services, support for women and children experiencing sexual violence, and educational work with men (Onyango and Majola, 2006; Treatment Action Campaign, 2004). It organised demonstrations, held doorstep discussions throughout the neighbourhood, raised the issue on TAC's weekly radio show and developed school-based programmes to work with young men. Such a campaign was consistent with the declared intentions of most HIV projects, at levels from the local to the international, to address HIV and gender issues in parallel – something that is recognised as crucial (Baylies and Bujra, 2001). It was also a 'rooted' response, instructively close to the local situation. It did not stay with the issue of HIV stigma focused on earlier in the epidemic, or restrict its address to women's lack of power, but made a more inclusive appeal to combat gender violence. Its generalising address called up some commonality between all residents, regardless of HIV status and gender, while still being able to recognise the specific interests of people who are HIV positive, and of women. This is collectively generated pragmatism, with future thinking built into it. For more formal and large-scale research and intervention programmes, it is an important kind of theory-in-action to learn from.

2   Researching HIV

The question of AIDS is an extremely important terrain of struggle and contestation. In addition to the people we know who are dying, or have died, or will, there are the many people dying who are never spoken of. How could we say that the question of AIDS is not also a question of who gets represented and who does not?

Stuart Hall, 1992

We should . . . welcome all the information retrieval in silenced areas that is taking place in anthropology, political science, history and sociology. Yet the assumption and construction of a consciousness or subject sustains such work and will, in the long run, cohere with the work of imperialist subject-constitution, mingling epistemic violence with the advancement of learning and civilisation and the subaltern women will be as mute as ever.

Gayatri Spivak, 1994 [1985]

Interviewer 1: So is there anything else that you think is important and that we haven't asked about?
Interviewer 3: *Ikhona enye into mhlawumbi obawela ukuthetha ngayo?*
    Is there anything else that you would like to talk about?
Ntomboxolo: *Ha ah, hayi nindibuzile and ndonelisekile. Ndonelisekile yimibuzo yenu enindibuze yona.*
No, you have asked me and I am satisfied. I am satisfied with the questions that you have asked me.

Interviewers and Ntoboxolo, Khayelitsha, June 2001

Situating the research

In 2001, I started doing interviews around Cape Town with people living with HIV with three research assistants, Nomvula Zenzile, Sabelo Mazibuko and Lumka Daniel. In 2003 and 2004, I reinterviewed some of our research participants. The interviews aimed to gather people's assessments of the support they had which helped them live with HIV, and the support they wished they had.

What did the interviewees in our research say about their participation, which for many constituted their most public declaration of themselves as

HIV positive subjects so far? One woman, who had talked only to her doctor about her diagnosis, told us she was very happy to have talked about HIV for the first time. Others, like Ntomboxolo in the interview segment quoted above, said simply that they were satisfied with the interview. Talking to us often seemed to be part of their more general plan to educate the world by demonstrating their own acceptance and understanding of being HIV positive. Several said they were pleased that people – in particular, people from outside their neighbourhood – were listening to what they had to say, at a time when they felt people with HIV were generally unheard. A few spontaneously indicated willingness to talk to other researchers or even the media. One, off tape, declared the importance of South Africans talking more openly about their experiences with HIV, 'like on *Ricki*' – the US *Ricki Lake* television talk show, broadcast widely in South Africa. Towards the end of interviews, some talked not about HIV at all, but about the more pressing need to get a job, or training, or to feed and educate their children.

Sometimes, participants got upset in the interviews, but wanted to continue. Everyone – except one person who was ill, and one young woman, interviewed on her own – talked at considerable length. Some interviews ended with people declaring they had said everything, others were constrained by the opening hours of the interview sites. We grew used to interviews that continued beyond their estimated time, those scheduled next politely putting their heads around the door to ask when we'd be ready, and at the end of a day, people sweeping up and meaningfully jangling the building's keys at us. Each time we left, people asked when we were coming back again so that they could get other people they knew to come and do the research. At each research site, there were people hovering around, asking questions, who had read the materials and who might have participated if we had returned again. Doing followup interviews on my return over the next couple of years was easy; people were keen to talk about what had or hadn't changed for them and for others. But it was hard to find the interviewees again. Interviewees diagnosed in relatively early stages of HIV disease, for instance many of the women diagnosed during pregnancy, were mostly well and had little contact with NGOs or clinics. Some interviewees had moved. Two, who had been ill when we first met, were known to have died.

As became clear in Chapter 1, this was a time of struggle and change for HIV positive people in the Western Cape. At the beginning of the research, MTCT – mother-to-child treatment to prevent HIV's transmission from positive pregnant women to their babies – was available for pregnant HIV positive women in the province, treatments for opportunistic infections were patchily accessible, and ARVs were being provided to small numbers. However, some interviewees were only receiving non-prescription pain-killers from their clinics. A disability grant could be obtained if HIV had made you severely ill or your CD4 count was dangerously low. Support groups were increasing in number; income generation groups were starting up. Openness about your HIV status was possible for a few people; some interviewees were campaigning for national MTCT and ARV access. By the research's end in 2004, a few interviewees had been taking ARVs for three or more years, and were dealing with long-term side-effects and the difficulties of combining chronic illness with paid work. Yet struggles for medical resources and against stigmatisation continued. Interviewees' HIV positive family members outside Cape Town rarely had ARV access. While some research participants were now completely open with relatives and friends, others remained concerned that even the healthy foods they wanted to cook might make their family suspect their status.

In this chapter, I want to situate our study, not just in relation to social science research, but also in relation to some of the artistic and activist work which inspired it, before describing how we conducted it. The chapter moves away from the book's initial concerns with the global and local shape of HIV epidemics to examine how different fields of action and research have tried to understand HIV, and how HIV research can learn from the pragmatic, reality- and future-orientated character of some of the most effective responses to the pandemic.

Activism, art and education as research

HIV is, Farmer suggests, 'the most spectacularly studied infection in human history' (1999: 50). However, its broader social significance has been surprisingly undertheorised in the social sciences. Early on, HIV activists, often themselves living with the virus, contributed importantly to understanding non-medical aspects of living with HIV and avoiding transmission. Lesbian feminists' and gay men's writing about safer sex established effective guidelines before HIV's viral nature had even been confirmed. Women living with HIV campaigned successfully for an expansion of the Centers for Disease Controls' AIDS definition to include symptoms experienced by women. Sex workers made key observations and interventions about the dangers of using nonoxynol-9 to inhibit HIV transmission. Organisations of people living with HIV in developed and developing countries campaigned persistently and effectively against stigmatisation and for education and treatment resources, in the face of often indifferent medical and political establishments. This kind of campaigning salutarily demonstrates the importance of pragmatism in the HIV field, for researchers as well as for activists. It was grounded in local contexts, but it also maintained a strong sense of the futures of effective treatment and prevention to which it aimed – a double-direction strategy that good HIV research also adopts.

Activism and research differ in important ways, too. Activists must often work within limited timeframes towards short-term goals that do not address all the issues social researchers might want to consider. For example, you cannot usefully campaign for ARVs and at the same time address the problems associated with decades-long ARV use. Disciplinary and institutional criteria of legitimacy can also seem clearer in social research than in activism. Activism's legitimacy is often disputed from 'above', as with the South African government officials' accusations that TAC is driven by interests other than those of the communities it claims to represent. Frequently, activism's claims are also contested from 'below'. In the late 1980s, groups within US ACT UP representing people of colour and women, started to organise separately from the main group, consisting largely of gay white men. A further group, seen by some as too committed to the medicalised 'norming' of HIV as a chronic, non-curable illness instead of to its eradication, split to become the Treatment Action Group.

Yet similar disputes happen within social research, revolving around the rigour of methods, the reliability of findings and the validity of the theories that make sense of those findings. It is hard for social researchers to produce clear results with agreed implications. The difficulty increases when health and social policymakers, in the middle of a pandemic, look to such results for answers. The debate over the HIV transmission-reducing effects of male circumcision is a recent example. This debate has to take account of regional, faith and ethnic variations in circumcision's practice, its cost and availability, its perceived health and sexual benefits, its relation to attitudes about religion, culture, modernity, and its possible risk-promoting effects if people see it as obviating safer sex or fewer partners – as well as its physiological effects on HIV transmission (Mattson *et al.*, 2005).

Literarature, art and media explored many HIV issues earlier than social research. There is a striking history of such work in the developed world, including playwriting and memoirs by gay men like Larry Kramer's *The Normal Heart* (1985), Paul Monette's *Borrowed Time* (1988), David Wojnarowicz's *Close to the Knives* (1991), Tony Kushner's *Angels in America* (1993); the writing of Edmund White (2000) in the US and Adam Mars-Jones (1993) in the UK; popular autobiographies by, for instance, Oscar Moore (1996); and work on women's place within the epidemic (ACT UP New York/Women and AIDS Book Group 1990, Rieder and Ruppelt 1989). Elisabeth Glaser's *In the Absence of Angels* (Glaser and Putnam, 1991) described the impact of AIDS on a Hollywood-successful white American family, in ways that brought the epidemic home for the first time to many middle-class heterosexual people in the US. Later, through the activities of her paediatric research foundation, Glaser linked this concern to expanded issues of HIV's impact on children in the developing world.

A varied array of fine art dealing with the pandemic, ranging from photographic portraiture to sculptural abstraction has been produced since the late 1980s.[1] Films such as *Silverlake Life* (Friedman and Joslin, 1993), *Blue* (Jarman, 1993) and *Longtime Companion* (Rene, 1990) provided important representations in the 1990s. *Philadelphia* (Demme, 1993), still the only big-budget Hollywood movie to address AIDS, proved revelatory for some US audiences despite presentations of illness, death and gay life by turns saccharine, melodramatic and conventionalised, that enraged some gay critics. Larry Kramer said of it, 'It's dishonest, it's often legally, medically and politically inaccurate, and it breaks my heart that I must say it's simply not good enough and I'd rather people not see it at all' (quoted in Corliss, 1994). Television representations expanded the reach of HIV images earlier and more widely, in the US through made-for-TV movies such as *An Early Frost* (Erman, 1985) and *Andre's Mother* (Reinisch, 1990). In the UK this happened predominantly through the long-term HIV positive character Mark Fowler in the popular television soap, *EastEnders*, whose storylines were written in consultation with HIV organisations and which provided most HIV information for young people in the late 1990s. The representational HIV citizenship created by ACT UP – starting with 'Silence=Death' posters, moving into street actions like 'die-ins' and same-sex 'kiss-ins', public art and civil disobedience – generated other engaged representations. The US AIDS Memorial Quilt, 45,000 commemorative panels, each measuring one by two metres, and its associated projects in 40 other countries across the world, are highly effective ways of inscribing HIV citizenship into public culture, as the 1996 display of the whole US Quilt in Washington, viewed by two million, demonstrated. A variety of critical social and political theories have developed around these activist, artistic and media representations, supporting and extending them,[2] and at the same time beginning to explore the global significance of the pandemic (Patton, 2002; Watney, 2000).

In Africa, representations of HIV have taken different forms. There are a small number of biographical and autobiographical texts, largely by white writers (for instance Cameron, 2005a; Levin, 2005) as well as some general texts designed for popular audiences (Mahlangu-Ngcobo, 2001). Southern Africa movies such as *States of Denial* (Epstein, 2002), *Shouting Silent* (Rosen and Sithole, 2002) and *Everyone's Child* (Dangaremgba, 1996) have been widely shown in the developing and developed world. We have already mentioned the televisual representations of HIV produced by *Soul City*. Youth-orientated television has also included, since 2002, an HIV positive puppet, Kami, in the South African version of *Sesame Street*. The controversial drama series *Yizo Yizo*, set in a township school, covered issues such as drugs, violence, rape and abuse as well as HIV, with bestselling soundtracks, a naturalistic visual style often criticised as too explicit about violence and sex, and fast editing reminiscent of music television (Barnett, 2004). Like *Soul City*, it managed to convey HIV information without forgetting that sex involves pleasure as well as health. Most TV and radio soaps have regular HIV-orientated storylines.[3] In Botswana, the Centres for Disease Control-sponsored *Rocky Road* radio serial serves as a *Soul City* parallel; there are many similar African and developing-world 'edutainment' soaps.[4] US talk shows seen in Africa, such as *Oprah* and *Ricki*, model open communication about intimate issues, and sometimes address HIV – but they are talking about a very different epidemic. More obviously relevant are South African-made shows like *Felicia*, an important early source of HIV information,[5] *Phat Joe Live*, a more youth-orientated show, and perhaps most influentially for English-language listeners, the *Tim Modise Show*, a radio phone-in which regularly debates controversial HIV issues such as the provision of treatment to pregnant HIV positive women, and the activities of Matthias Rath. HIV now frequently appears at least as a minor character in contemporary South African fiction (Ndebele, 2004) and in visual art. There is in addition a large body of photojournalism which has had strong international impact.[6] Many groups of people living with HIV have developed art and craft products income-generation projects which represent HIV, either directly, through for instance the red ribbon symbol, sold as beaded brooches all over South Africa, or metaphorically, in pieces such as the Durban Siyazama group's beaded crucified figures of women wearing AIDS ribbons.[7]

HIV issues also have a strong presence in African popular music and song that has no direct parallels in the developed world, though it appears in other developing-world contexts (Farmer, 1999). Sometimes this involves concerts 'for' HIV, such as the Mandela-organised 4664 event. HIV, like other political issues, is also sung and spoken about publically and frequently – though not always positively – by musicians.[8] Locally, again following political traditions in many parts of the continent, HIV activist groups often produce their own songs to educate and motivate people at meetings and demonstrations. In Uganda, TASO use music throughout their educational activities (Cohen, 2004). TAC's young women activists in the early 2000s, campaigning for MTCT, made up a song about getting pregnant and having a healthy baby, complete with vivid 'pregnant stomach' gestures and dancing.

Frequently, HIV-related art and media foreground the unpredictability and complexity of HIV, both personal and collective. These are characteristics of the pandemic which social research may gloss over, and that attention to HIV-related art and media can helpfully point up. The AIDS Memorial Quilt is an example of such difficult personal and social negotiations. Seen as morbid by some people living with the virus, and an appropriate kind of mourning and remembering by others, it is so diverse as to be hard to generalise about. Sometimes, just making a memorial panel – like just talking about HIV – can have large significance. As Stuart Hall says, in the quotation at the beginning of this chapter, many people living within the pandemic have not spoken, been spoken of, or been represented in any other way. Art can be a form of surrogate speech for people affected by the virus and not represented, or not heard. Yet art is at times too particular really to 'represent' the pandemic, and its claims to do so may be contested. As artists began to make work about HIV in the US, ACT UP insisted on the significance of the political ownership of such art, by both producers and audience (Crimp and Ralston, 1990), in response to images they viewed as idealised, tragic or simply unengaged with the realities of the epidemic. Today, photojournalistic images of Africans, usually women, living with HIV that appear on western television screens, mostly at the time of World AIDS Day, tend to carry a similarly emotive yet pessimistic charge. The most widely seen imagery of a different kind is probably the photography of Gideon Mendel, which includes framings chosen by his portrait subjects; self-descriptions, many of which parallel the accounts given by our interviewees and summarised in the next chapter; and at times panoramas of people's life circumstances.[9] This work avoids pathos and fatality, helpfully addresses the cultural phenomenology of HIV, and at the same time manages to pay attention to the social structures that inflect people's lives with the virus. This is a balancing act that social research also needs to pursue.

HIV education and prevention work provide a large number of confusing, though useful, indications of directions for social research. Campaigns like loveLife, *Soul City* and Khomanani, described in the previous chapter, operate across international, governmental, private and civil society institutions. Suspended between research, politics and media practice, and bringing with them stories of qualified success and almost complete failure, they, too, are hard to generalise about. The conclusions that can most consistently be drawn from such campaigns are that stakeholder involvement, and careful planning and evaluation, are important. The most apparently successful productions, such as *Soul City* and *Rocky Road*, also suggest the importance of flexible and diverse approaches, using | various media, and collaborating with concurrent community interventions (Galavotti *et al.*, 2001; Papa *et al.*, 2001; Soul City/MarkData, 2005). Social research about HIV, often constrained by narrow methods and limited community involvement, can learn from these approaches.

The web of difficulties involved in community- rather than media-based HIV awareness and education is somewhat different. Cathy Campbell's (2003) *Letting Them Die?* is an influential clarification of the problems. Campbell's book assesses an HIV prevention intervention in a mining settlement near Johannesburg, a well-designed project focused on miners, sex workers and young people, with other stakeholders from inside and outside the settlement involved in its design and execution. The project avoided the individual or the broad-brush 'community' focus of much work on HIV knowledge and decision-making, and focused instead on building 'social capital' – social identities, networks, and action (Putnam, 2000)[10] – within and between social groupings. During the project, youth and sex worker peer educators became knowledgeable and empowered; there was, therefore, some increase in 'bonding' social capital, links within social groups. HIV knowledge also generally improved, but condom use did not increase and HIV and other STI rates continued to rise. There was little increase in 'bridging' social capital, links between social groupings, including groups that are hierarchically differentiated. What went wrong? First, miners' conceptualisations of a 'risky' masculinity associated with the high risks of mining, made condom risk reduction hard to achieve. Second, 'sex workers' did not themselves adopt this identity – unlike in some successful HIV projects among sex workers, where there is often pre-existing activism. The women did not operate collectively to demand condom use, as workers in successful projects do (Cornish, 2004); there were no economic alternatives available to them. Third, many young people continued to see themselves as immune, or were in situations of economic dependency which made it hard to take on HIV messages, and did not identify with the peer educators. There were institutional problems also. Despite official endorsement, the mining organisations continued to treat HIV as best addressed simply by providing information. Schoolteachers were not fully supportive, experiencing the difficulties adults frequently encounter in talking about HIV, sexuality, and gendered identities more generally (Burns, 2002; Matthews *et al.*, 2006; Morrell *et al;*, 2002). Settlement residents' participation in project management was low, due to lack of time and skills. There were problems with stakeholders' involvement. Their commitment was uneven, their power highly differentiated and their accountability structures underdeveloped. Medical and other professional hierarchies' interests interfered with the participatory commitments of the project. The research team also had to negotiate with informal but armed male leaders of the settlement for access.

Campbell draws some useful conclusions from this project, suggesting that HIV initiatives of this kind should be building bonding and bridging social capital, links within and between social groupings; should be peer-focused and peer-initiated if possible; and should involve all relevant stakeholders, plus external as well as internal change agents, thus working in both top-down and bottom-up directions. Her account demonstrates how difficult it is to deliver HIV 'empowerment', even on some quite specific and modest 'social capital' measures, unless a comprehensive programme is embarked on that addresses economic and social change issues generally, as well as HIV, and that does not rely on an over-simple notion of 'community' (Barnett and Whiteside, 2006). Even then, 'empowerment' does not spill over from one area into another very easily. 'Social capital'-building, even if it can be achieved, is unlikely to work without political strategy (Edwards and Foley, 1998). As Campbell says:

> the extent to which people have the ability to adopt new sexual behaviours and to safeguard their health is dramatically constrained by the degree to which social circumstances support or enable them in these challenges.
>
> (2003: 184)

In our interviews, research participants' address to HIV issues frequently seemed to depend on broader social changes, and it was a relationship of which they were very aware. For example, women who were part of recently provided MTCT programmes often described these programmes – particularly but not only the negative test results of their babies – as allowing them to disclose to their families, not just as HIV positive, but as living healthily, safely and 'positively' with the virus. They also, correctly, saw these programmes as harbingers of new treatment opportunities and group support projects for themselves.

Social research

Social research around HIV has focused on prevention-oriented attitudes and behaviours, and to a lesser extent, especially in the developing world, on factors that enable people to live healthily with HIV. Influential early work, for instance, addressed peer network models of behaviour change, HIV stigma, effective counselling practices (Bor *et al.*, 1993; Herek, 1990; Kelly *et al.*, 1991;) and the specificity of women's and people of colour's concerns within the epidemic (for instance, Amaro, 1988; Mays and Cochran, 1988; Richardson, 1987). A parallel strand of work explored broader frameworks of social understanding around the pandemic (Aggleton and Homans, 1988).[11] Today, large numbers of researchers and academics in psychology, sociology and anthropology contribute to global and local HIV prevention and treatment services, at levels from neighbourhood clinics and community-based organisations (CBOs), through to multinational projects such as the behavioural science elements of the Centers for Disease Control's Global AIDS Programme.

The success of such work is hard to evaluate, implicated with other factors and much contested. For in the case of HIV, social research's complexities are particularly strong. First, it has to address the powerful cultural as well as individual and social aspects of the epidemics. Campbell's study, for instance, addressed the lack of a sex worker 'identity' among the women studied, a microcultural resource which among organised groups of sex workers in India, for instance, can help communities deal with HIV (Cornish, 2004). The interview project this book describes aimed to examine what public representations – not just of HIV – were available, and how they were used in people's personal repertoires for representing HIV – some of which may be constraining, and some helpful.

Our research was based on individuals' accounts of their HIV experiences. This type of research around HIV also has to be approached cautiously. Concepts of self and identity current in mainstream western social psychology are not always useful in relation to HIV. Campbell (2003) points critically to the individual focus of much work on HIV knowledge and decision making; Farmer (1999: 98) notes the unmerited causal power that psychological factors such as 'low self-esteem' and 'denial' acquire in many accounts of the pandemic. Individual-centred work often fails to look at higher structural levels, for instance, the criteria of national and international organisations (Van Vlaenderen and Neves, 2004), which can significantly affect how research participants respond to questions. It also downplays social relations among families and friends. The questions about HIV 'support' posed in this research needed to investigate the complex network of social relations within which HIV is lived. To avoid making presumptions about the individual impact of HIV, our research did not solicit personal stories, or assume such stories were highly significant. It did not even assume that HIV was central to people's lives or their self-representations.

The inappropriateness of an individual-centred approach is particularly obvious in developing-world situations where social networks may be both more personally foregrounded, and more conventionally accepted as a resource. I am not here making an argument for Afrocentric (King *et al.*, 1976; Jones, 1972) or more generally sociocentric (Shweder, 1991) conceptualisations of identity, or for the notion of an 'African' interconnected or relational self (Ogbonnaya, 1994), although some of these concepts are certainly relevant to this research. Since 'culture', including 'African' culture, is not a homogeneous or static thing, we might expect more variability and fluidity than such concepts imply (Ratele, 2004).

Contemporary social science is less likely to apply western conceptions of 'identity' (Kiguwa, 2004) to HIV issues than a decade ago. There is a considerable body of work that explicitly criticises such concepts. It seemed appropriate, in this research, to keep the notion of fixed 'identity' in question, holding onto the possibility both of addressing it, as Stuart Hall (1994) suggests, as fluid and changing 'identifications', and of remembering Spivak's often-appropriated notion of 'strategic essentialism' (1990) in order to describe effective subjects. At times, Spivak's (1994 [1985]) notion of the subaltern, unspeaking subject does seem relevant to developed-world discourse about HIV which largely silences HIV positive developing-world citizens. However, as the quotation at the beginning of this chapter indicates, the 'subaltern' is not some kind of acceptable charitable focus for research. This research was done at a time when many people had begun to speak about HIV, and were fighting for new modes of HIV subjecthood. What seemed important, in the face of the sudden and large-scale phenomenon of South African epidemic, was to document participants' own representations as theories in themselves, putting other theories of HIV and subjectivity to one side.

Much social research around HIV, being publicly funded and policy orientated, has short-term instrumental aims such as discovering what factors increase condom use or produce ARV treatment adherence. It necessarily neglects other potentially significant aspects of the research context, including many aspects of support. Some developed-world studies have found social support to be important for HIV positive people's long-term physical and mental health as well as their short-term state (Green, 1993; Knowlton *et al.*, 2004; MacMahon *et al.*, 2000; Song and Ingram, 2002). Family and social network support is often addressed separately from support groups (Davison *et al.*, 2000; Walch *et al.*, 2006). There is remarkably little South African work on support, except in relation to particular treatment programmes (Skogmar *et al.*, 2006; Stenson *et al.*, 2005) or transmission risk reduction.

Social support is not easy to define, and causal aspects of its relation to health generally, as well as to HIV, are unclear (Green, 1993; Sarason *et al.*, 1990). Most work on social support operates with predefined support categories, and quantifies responses. These procedures introduce some rigour to an important but undertheorised field. In social research around HIV, moreover, policy demands mean that quantitative work is usually preferred. This means that qualitative studies of what people say about HIV in their lives are few; qualitative material tends to be used to illustrate quantitative findings. To focus not just on qualitative content but on stories of HIV might seem, however engaging, an irrelevant 'footnote' to serious research. Such work appears, indeed, mainly in literary and artistic representations of HIV. Yet 'support' is a concept that evokes a wide network of meanings, easily connecting with important social and cultural formations around HIV that are unlikely to be measured adequately by quantifiable, fixed-response categories.

The idea of conducting qualitative research around HIV support in South Africa, using the relatively open procedure of semi-structured interviews, came from my experiences conducting similar research over the previous decade with people infected or affected by HIV in Britain, some of whom have now taken part in four interviews. This study has, like similar others, found that participants take time in interviews to explain their strategies for living positively with HIV positive status, and use particular representational resources that seem to support these strategies (Carricaburu and Pierret, 1995; Ciambrone, 2001; Ezzy, 2000; Squire, 1999, 2003, 2006). Impetus for the South African research also came from helping conduct HIV support groups in New Jersey in the late 1980s and early 1990s, an experience that alerted me to the strong and unpredictable significance that different forms of support have for people living with HIV in varying health and social circumstances. The South African research, rather than eliciting clear evaluations of specific support resources, aimed to explore people's own frames of understanding and evaluating support, as they defined it, for living with HIV.

Another important question for social science HIV research concerns the relations between researchers and participants. How participant-centred can research usefully be? My research did not make many assumptions about what activities or ways of talking were better, beyond viewing positively those discourses and practices that research participants themselves assessed as keeping them healthy and improving their lives. In interpreting the interviews, I also assumed a weak correlation between modes of talk and modes of action (Plummer, 1995) – a correlation explored through the content of participants' talk, and its structure in relation to the structure of talk in everyday life.

More prescriptively, the research assumed the value of safe sex even if participants did not practise it; and of medical treatment shown to be effective for HIV and HIV-related conditions even if participants did not want it. This was the hierarchised limit of its participant-centredness. It did not affect how

I and the research assistants did the interviews. But it meant that if participants asked about medical or other help, we referred them to mainstream public and accredited NGO provision. Moreover, in interpreting the interviews, I operated with conventional medical criteria about safe and unsafe behaviours, and what treatments are appropriate at different HIV disease stages. As the researcher, I judge my stance the correct one, and have the institutional power to represent it as such. In this particular case, it can be argued for medically, socially and politically, and the evolving popular history of South African responses to the epidemic also tends to endorse it.

Differences between researchers and research participants operate in many other ways – not necessarily always negatively – when the research involves black South African participants, mostly unemployed or in relatively low-paying jobs; black South African research assistants, well educated and working in universities; and a white British researcher from a UK university.[12] Our gender (female, in three cases) was not incidental to what people told us. Lumka's and Sabelo's young age clearly affected younger interviewees' relationships with them. Nomvula, Lumka and Sabelo were seen as understanding aspects of Xhosa culture that could in some cases be mentioned and in some cases need not be talked about because they were assumed known. Such things might need to be explained to me, or might usefully be left out. From interviewees' explicit comments, I was most saliently perceived as white, although sometimes my being English, or at least not South African, seemed to affect how people framed their accounts. So did my being around five to ten years older than most interviewees – and even my being a parent. My daughter was in a few interviews, playing with the babies and toddlers the women interviewees brought along.

Spending only short periods of time in South Africa, and speaking just one of its 11 recognised languages, I have a very incomplete understanding of the South African epidemic and the historical and political circumstances that surround it. Despite wide comprehension of English, and the power of English-language HIV representations in South Africa, being restricted to English biased the project. More broadly, while all perspectives are, of course, limited, mine is, I think, objectively more limited than understandings held by many South Africans working on HIV issues, particularly those who are themselves HIV positive or who are – as are most South Africans today – surrounded by HIV concerns. I cannot reach their kind of intimate and joined-up understandings.

Given the complex and dramatic power relations operating in HIV research in the developing world, and my own positioning within them as a white western academic, I could be almost endlessly reflexive about this research. To ignore the power relations of interviews may implicitly reproduce them. When, for instance, I quote Ntomboxolo at the beginning of this chapter, as 'satisfied' with her interview, it is important to read this quote in the context of the two quotes about silencing and subaltern status that come beforehand – and that Ntomboxolo's words do not erase at all.

However, to concentrate on dominant power relations may subsume research participants into them, as if they cannot speak or act outside them. The powerful significance of HIV in South Africa to some degree overwhelmed interactions between myself and the interviewees, as indicated by interviewees' own concerns about the wider audiences for their words. My interpretations control the material to a large extent, but they are partial, contestable and clearly not definitive.

One way to address the hierarchy and differences between researcher and participants is to conduct research that tries to undo them. Participatory Action Research (PAR) sets out to develop research strategies collaboratively with participants instead of imposing them. However, 'participation' may be much less important for research participants than some more concrete requirements – for example, in the case of many of our interviewees, treatment access. PAR is ineffective in a vacuum; it has to be connected up to relevant, implemented policies, and this is difficult to achieve in a situation of national economic difficulty and global inequality. In the case of HIV, relatively short-term and obviously non-local researchers such as myself may pose confidentiality problems and even material dangers by demanding 'participation'. It is also impossible for such researchers to 'participate' fully or combine research's aims with community activist ones (Sigoga and Tso Modipa, 2004). They remain hierarchically privileged outsiders, however carefully the research is formulated (Campbell, 2003). Even the most thoroughly 'community'-based research projects often last too little time for researchers really to understand local knowledge (Sigoga and Tso Modipa, 2004), and may end up reinforcing existing power structures – for instance by concentrating on the most powerful community members as informants and gatekeepers. Such projects may also – like other highly particular qualitative research – become too imbricated in specificities to allow generalisation (MacLeod, 2004).[13]

The word 'community', which appears often in HIV research aimed at inclusiveness, is itself problematic, and is used cautiously in this book. It can be both totalising and oversimplifying. In the South African context it is racialised: 'communities' are where non-whites live (Sigoga and Tso Modipa, 2004). In addition, neighbourhoods in South Africa, despite having strong local identities, are heterogeneous and in flux, particularly in the areas of rapid and recent urbanisation where most of our research participants lived. To call such neighbourhoods 'communities' may overestimate their commonalities. Even if the term 'community' is used broadly, to connote ideas and histories held in common within neighbourhood-based social networks, it might assume too much similarity. 'Community' is also often used to refer to other forms of, for instance, health, professional, religious or other chosen, 'elective' (Weeks, 1985) commonalities. Thus 'community' is deployed as a marker of a very wide range of social associations – of the kind 'social capital' theorists are interested in, for instance – as well as of productive actions; and at times, of constraint and homogenisation. This book uses the term little, preferring a pragmatic concept of citizenship: a set of different linkages, established at varying levels from the neighbourhood to the transnational, and involving criticism as well as association (Mouffe, 1992; Walzer, 1983).[14] The book does at times use the term 'community' in a geographical sense, although our interviewees clearly indicated the limits to neighbourhood commonality.

The people who are really doing PAR are those within a specific neighbourhood who – like some of our research participants – are consciously engaged in HIV education and prevention, either as part of locally based community or activist projects, or informally, by talking with their friends. As NGOs and CBOs now recognise, they have a great deal of implicit knowledge that they can usefully render explicit.[15] Such knowledge can be generalised by connecting with other, similar projects, as happens already, to some degree, between South African HIV programmes. This is the kind of research that can best work against the 'mute' subaltern status of which Spivak (1994: 90) writes.

The research described here was not set up as PAR, but operated at one remove, documenting what people thought was working in the HIV services available to them, as well as in non-HIV-related services, and in family and friendship support networks. However, the research still had to consider many of the problems noted in the PAR literature around participation and 'community', the generality of findings, and action. For instance, it distanced itself from medical and social service institutions and authority; but this separation was not always taken much note of by research participants. At times, interviewees addressed us as channels to media awareness or practical help, rather than as researchers. This was logical, in contexts where middle-class whites and blacks, if not medical professionals or teachers, generally appeared only as journalists, pastors, NGO donors or officers of local government, and where resource shortages made any possibility of practical help important to pursue. The research was participant-directed, focused on interviewees' own words; but it was guided by a topic list of areas for interview discussion. It was structured to include feedback and some followup interviews; but the realities of participants' complicated and resource-limited lives made these hard to implement fully.

Contemporary social science research around HIV is closer to activist concerns than in the past. In a pandemic now widely recognised to be shaped by gendered power relations, the relationship to activism includes important ties to feminist work. The meaning of 'feminism' and even the term itself is contested in many developing-world contexts. Sometimes it is dismissed as a western imposition; at other times feminism and its variants, including African feminisms and womanisms, are debated (Kiguwa, 2004; Mama, 2001; Ogundipe-Leslie, 1994).[16] South Africa has a long history of resistance to women's 'triple oppression' as black, working class and female (Kuzwayo, 2004 [1985]; Russell, 1989); of women's political action; and of debates about gender within the anti-apartheid movement and later, the ANC government. The country has a long-established legacy of racially and economically diverse women's groups and publications, such as the ANC Women's League, the Black Sash, the journals *Speak!* and *Agenda*, writers such as the late Ellen Kuzwayo, Bessie Head, Nadine Gordimer and Antje Krog, and major political figures like Winnie Madikizela-Mandela, Albertina Sisulu, Frene Ginwala, Mamphela Ramphele – and the ex-health minister, Nkosozama Zuma herself.

Today there is, as the previous chapter indicated, extensive work being done on gender and HIV in South Africa, particularly around prevention and education. To a large extent, such work reflects current international approaches to gender issues through 'mainstreaming', a process of considering and acting against gender inequalities in every area of people's lives, formulated at the Beijing Fourth International Conference on Women (United Nations, 1997; see also Rounaq, 1995). In South Africa, as more generally, shortcomings of this approach have included addresses to gender in policy, not practice; and tokenistic inclusions of women in decision-making (Hassim, 2004). In HIV organisations, such marginalisation can involve, for instance, declarations about the importance of addressing violence against women, and women's unequal power to negotiate safer sex, that are unconnected to action; or a concentration of women at organisations' lower levels, and their tokenistic presence higher up. Women are integral to most HIV organisations in South Africa. Nevertheless, it often happens that organisations dependent on women to deliver their services and give them ideas about what is and is not working, and what to do next, do not include them fully in policy-making. These failings may easily be replicated in research. I was aware, for instance, that talking to volunteer interviewees, in a 'community' not our own, about a gender-sensitive topic, would not always deliver a fully gender-aware perspective, even though I was talking mostly to women. Yet for researchers to operate with their own 'gender-transformative' agenda, especially in a short-term, externally organised project, is a disruptive imposition. The best way to enable such an agenda seemed to be to allow the women and men we interviewed to set out their own understandings of, for instance, relationships and safer sex in talking to us, and for us to provide appropriate referrals and to frame our questions in ways that allowed, without requiring, talk about gender issues.

Mainstreaming was also meant to include women in human rights work previously slanted towards men's rights (Cook, 1994). Many argue that it has failed in this respect (Charlesworth, 2005) and suggest a more specific address to 'women's human rights' (Oloka-Onyango and Tamale, 1995). In the HIV field, this address now appears in international organisations' awareness of how gender-based violence relates to the pandemic, and their interest in moving towards women-orientated prevention technologies such as microbicides and the female condom. South Africa's legal guarantee, in the context of the HIV epidemic, of young women's right not to be tested for virginity,[17] also responds to the demand that women's rights be 'mainstreamed' within human rights (South Africa Commission for Gender Equality and South Africa Human Rights Commission, 2001). However, the demand is less well met in other areas of HIV policy, for instance, in perceived government reluctance to address the connections between HIV and gender-based violence, or to support ARV treatment for women who have been raped. The Khayelitsha campaign, in the wake of Lorna Mlofana's murder, made local access to treatment of this kind a priority, and South African advocacy organisations for physically and sexually abused women are now numerous and high profile. South African HIV research has also addressed these issues comprehensively (Jewkes and Abrahams, 2002). Specifically raising them in our project would, again, have been an imposition. Again, we enabled and supported their discussion if interviewees themselves raised them, and provided suitable sources of support where relevant.

For research exploring the meanings of the epidemic in a specific place and time, the above might be overgeneral frameworks. They might, for instance, overlook important microstructures of gendered power in young people's understandings of HIV and their lives, like the relations young women have with men who support them economically and with whom they have sex (Morrell *et al.*, 2002; Selikow *et al.*, 2002). Some of our young women interviewees told of 'boyfriends' they loved who were also vital for their economic support. Framing these relationships as coercive or even transactional would not have described them adequately. Campaigns like the Khayelitsha response to Lorna Mlofana's murder, which mobilised men as well as women against gender violence, also point to new approaches to masculinities in the context of African HIV epidemics (Onyango and Majola, 2006). Some of our male interviewees' reformulations of their lives and relationships in relation to HIV exemplified such moves.

My own predominantly first-world knowledge of feminist debates and actions was of limited help in preparing for this research. The project considered gender where it was raised explicitly as a topic, or where there was clearly gendered content in the interviews, even if these occurrences did not relate obviously to existing work around gender and HIV. As with 'psychology', however, it left 'feminism' in the background, rather than pre-deciding its significance, and moved participants' own representations to the foreground. A new and diverse phenomenon like the HIV pandemic requires feminist research, as well as social research, to adapt to the new circumstances and if necessary, change character.

The research presented here is a highly specific picture of the support that people had and wanted for living with HIV, in a particular time and place. It eschews universalising theoretical frameworks for theoretical pragmatism. Its procedural emphasis on people speaking about HIV, matched local, medical and political concerns with acceptance, disclosure and openness, as well as interviewees' own interests in this matter. Yet adopting Farmer's (1999) suggestions about research on infectious diseases, the research tries to be '*dynamic, systemic* and *critical*' (43; emphasis in original). It is attentive to higher levels of context, such as that of contemporary medical and religious discourses, and to national and transnational political contexts. It addresses the popular and personal representations that are key phenomena in this pandemic. These concerns give it some wider significance for social-scientific work on HIV epidemics with similar epidemiological, historical or socioeconomic conditions.[18]

Doing the research

The research was conducted mainly in three township areas around Cape Town. Inhabitants of the townships are almost all black African people, mostly Xhosa-speaking, and HIV rates are high, thought in 2004 to be around 27 per cent among pregnant women (Shaikh *et al.*, 2006). The townships include some middle-class housing; many more modest, working-class houses; and large informal settlements of one-room dwellings constructed from wood, corrugated iron, plastic and cardboard, often far from clinics and with little infrastructure. Unemployment is generally high – well over 50 per cent in informal settlements (Ndingaye, 2005). Khayelitsha, with 400,000 inhabitants at the 2001 census (a conservative estimate), is the biggest and also the newest township near Cape Town, dating from the 1980s, with the largest percentage of informal settlement dwellings. Many people living in informal settlements have arrived relatively recently, often from rural areas with less extensive HIV education and testing. However, Western Cape township HIV education and services are relatively good. This service level was a prerequisite for doing a study of HIV 'support' which cannot practically or ethically be discussed if it is not known about or available.

Western Cape HIV testing rates, particularly antenatally, were also relatively high, bolstered by the province's rollout of MTCT which drew in women who knew or suspected they were HIV positive.[19] A few of our interviewees had indeed travelled while pregnant from the Eastern Cape, taking cheap, exhausting and circuitous routes to get to Cape Town and obtain the best possible care for their babies. Such microstrategies of HIV knowledge and action are highly instructive about people's commitment and creativity when dealing with HIV in under-resourced settings.

We recruited interviewees through interested NGOs, CBOs, counsellors and support group facilitators, and chain referral from previous interviewees. We had meetings and telephone discussions with relevant groups and their 'gatekeeper' representatives first, to explain the research and find out if they wanted to be involved.[20] We also got valuable feedback on what these groups wanted to learn from the research. The three gatekeepers most involved with these discussions, and in closest contact with research participants, were interviewed themselves.

Initially we conducted 37 interviews, with 29 female and eight male research participants. Interviews were conducted either by me in English, or by myself and a research assistant, partly or wholly in Xhosa. Of the research assistants, Sabelo Mazibuko was a University of Cape Town undergraduate student; Lumka Daniel, a graduate student at UCT; and Nomvula Zenzile worked as an interviewer for local NGOs. In 2003–4, I visited the research sites again, carried out English-language interviews with NGO and CBO gatekeepers and some interviewees, and made one return visit to a support group. In this way, followup interviews were conducted with eight of the original sample. Some interviewees were known to have moved away from Cape Town. Sadly, though unsurprisingly, two were known to have died. The 12 interviewees using MTCT groups in 2001 were least easy to contact. Many, tested and diagnosed because of pregnancy not illness, were not using HIV services. Some were said still to be involved with HIV services as peer mentors on the 'mothers to mothers to be' programmes now running alongside MTCT; in income generation groups doing beadwork or metal-work; or as home carers for other HIV positive people. One MTCT support group facilitator said she frequently saw ex-members of her groups shopping or hurrying to work, and they would simply smile at each other.

A few interviews were done at the University of Cape Town, where I was visiting the Department of Psychology, but most were conducted in the offices of CBOs or NGOs. These were people's preferred venues; no one wanted to be interviewed at home. Though not performed in the context of research participants' daily lives, interview contexts were therefore close to the HIV realities of their lives. From the low levels of disclosure reported by many interviewees, the loss of confidentiality involved by a strange person or people, one white, visiting people's homes, would have been problematic.

Of 34 HIV positive interviewees, 22 had been diagnosed in 2000 or 2001 – including 19 women – with the rest spaced out through the 1990s, dating back to 1992. Of the 12 women on MTCT programmes, only one reported being previously diagnosed. Women participate more in HIV support services, and at earlier stages of HIV illness, in South Africa, as elsewhere; there were more women in the mixed-gender HIV support groups we contacted. Out of seven HIV positive men we interviewed, all but one had experienced HIV-related illness. Most of our non-MTCT female inter-viewees also had HIV illness histories, however, so with these small numbers, no clear gender differences in illness and service use among the non-MTCT interviewees emerged.

Women tend to be over-represented in much sexual and reproductive health research, and in HIV prevalence research. However, qualitative HIV research has focused mostly on men in the developed world. The over-representation of women in the group was therefore an advantage. Women are often said to be more likely to volunteer for interview research. However, when mixed-gender support groups came to hear of this research, men tended to volunteer first. This may have been partly related to men's greater comfort with speaking English, which might also reflect higher educational levels. Once one man from a group had volunteered, though, this opened the way for other men who did not choose an English-language interview. Early-volunteering female interviewees also included those most confident about speaking English and perhaps, those most educated. However, women who had been in contact with HIV services for a long time also volunteered quickly.

All interviewees were black African and had English or Xhosa as their most-used language. Participants varied in age from late teens to forties, and in class, from middle-class, college- or university-educated, to interviewees who had matriculated from secondary school, to many interviewees who reported not finishing secondary school.[21] Types of medical support used included state clinics, private doctors and traditional healers, in various combinations. HIV illness ranged from asymptomatic to stage 4 HIV illness (World Health Organisation, 2005).

Interviewees were drawn to the project by a number of motivations: through activist engagement; a personal sense of wanting to talk openly but anonymously about HIV, for their own or others' benefit; as part of a friendship network; for the accompanying honorarium; or for several of these reasons. People who were not outgoing, practised in talking about HIV, or motivated by personal or political agendas, and who might not otherwise have volunteered for interview research, could be engaged initially by the fee or by a friend's persuasion; but all the participants talked at considerable length once involved. Many interviewees volunteered before they knew about the fee. Some said they were glad that we had come to do the study as they thought the epidemic they were living through had been forgotten by the richer and more powerful people outside their local neighbourhoods. Others declared they wanted to participate because they themselves wanted to talk about HIV, or in order to help others with the condition. Some indicated they volunteered simply because they had heard from previous interviewees that the interview was unproblematic and interesting to do.

Participants were interviewed individually (16) and in groups (21) of two (one group), three (five groups) and four (one group). These were friendship groupings, usually originating from support groups. They allowed peer support to participants who were initially nervous about the interviews. Other researchers have found (Frosh *et al.*, 2003) that while more ambiguous and disclosing self-characterisations emerge in individual interviews, groups address a broader range of issues and engage in debates. Our small-group interviewees spent less time on 'personal' issues such as sexual and parent-child relationships, and sometimes echoed each others' responses, but they also usefully disagreed, for instance, over the value of local versus non-local support groups, whether nurses or doctors were sympathetic about HIV, and how and when to disclose to your children. Individual interviews did indeed feature more uncertainties and conflicts – but mainly because interviewees least in touch with HIV services were recruited for individual interviews. Pam, for instance, had support from her family, but no regular medical treatment, and knew no openly positive people except for one dying friend.

Hers was the interview that focused most on ambiguities about condom use and status disclosure to partners. However, group interviews also contained ambiguities, for instance, when disagreements were indicated but not explicitly addressed – over, for example, the role of particular facilitators in support groups. They demonstrated, too, some interesting convergences – for instance, about the difficulties of funeral costs, the appetite-stimulating effects of multivitamins, the rudeness of non-specialist medical staff, and the demand for ARVs – that did not emerge so strongly in individual interviews. Groups gave an opportunity to listen, providing exemplars for people who wanted to talk but found this hard to do in a one-to-one interview. At times, also, the groups performed the supportive functions they were telling us about, enacting encouragement and advice at the same time as describing them. Women from MTCT programmes, for instance, collectively described the stories they had developed to explain why they were not breast-feeding, and group members often provided collaborative accounts of healthy nutrition for the HIV positive. These performances were powerful demon-strations of research participants' commitment to building 'interpretive communities' (Plummer, 1995) around HIV.

Other reasons for the small-group interviews were logistic and political. Several support groups volunteered, not as individuals, as we had predicted, but almost as a whole. There was no fair way to select individuals from these groups, and people could not be asked to return another day since this necessitated long, expensive and health-compromising travel. When joint interviews were clarified as a possibility, we also had many volunteers from women on MTCT programmes who were previously hesitant about partici-pating. This structure, like the fee, thus produced a broader range of interviewees than might otherwise have participated.

Interviews started with a detailed consent form describing the research's purpose and destinations and interviewees' rights to change anything or limit or stop participating, offering transcripts, and specifying that interviews would be confidential, anonymised in transcription, and the transcripts archived. Interviewees could also choose an alternative name by which the transcripts would refer to them.[22] It was important to discuss the materials as well as allowing time for reading, especially since full literacy could not be assumed. Interviewees came to the study with a variety of ideas about it, garnered from previous interviewees, research gatekeepers' different accounts, and their own perceptions of the leaflet announcing it, but also in some cases from their experiences of HIV research more generally, and more importantly perhaps, from their perceptions of HIV representations in the media, their experiences of HIV services and their experiences of family, friends' and community reactions to HIV.

We offered refreshments – juice and muffins – to participants, who had no other such provision available and were in many cases extending an already-long day at a nearby clinic, support group or CBO to take part in the research. The refreshments were very popular, and an important part of setting an open and warm tone for the interviews, something which, as we shall see, the participants valued in the HIV support they received generally.

We told participants we hoped to gather their opinions of support in their own terms, rather than in terms of specific categories, and that we planned to produce a research-dedicated archive of people's accounts of their strategies for living with HIV. Early on, it became clear that many people wanted to use the interviews to talk about their HIV experiences generally, and wanted their interviews preserved. The requirement set by some ethics committees to destroy data after the research would have had very negative effects on this project.

We interviewed participants about their experiences of a broad range of different kinds of support for living with HIV. This openness did not seem problematic. As in most qualitative interviewing, participants were occasionally concerned that they had gone off topic; we then reiterated our opening expression of interest in what *they* thought were relevant elements of HIV support. A few remarked that they appreciated being able to speak at length and in their own terms, having had previous more structured research experiences. 'Support' was a well-understood term even for interviewees who spoke little English, in part through the familiarity of many with the term 'support group'. In translation, the research assistants rendered 'support' as 'help', 'encouragement', or as a word close to 'support' in English, that has connotations with physically holding something up. Sometimes, 'support' appeared as an English-derived, Xhosalised term, a common practice in South Africa, where languages that are in contact often acquire vocabulary from each other. There was considerable overlap between practical and psychological meanings in the ways interviewees used the words, although occasionally, 'encouragement' or 'talking' was contrasted with practical 'help'.

The interviews used open-ended questions and some reflecting back to check understanding. They covered topics that previous HIV support research (Green, 1993) and pilot interviews suggested might be significant: traditional and western medicine, counselling, social services, the voluntary sector, family, friendship, religion, community and government. However, topic choice and duration came predominantly from interviewees. If they wanted to talk at length about particular support elements we did not press them to divert to others, even if for logistical reasons the interview was drawing to a close. Some interviewees chose to tell the story of their lives with HIV. We did not interrupt, though we asked about areas that had not been covered at the end. We did not pursue HIV 'career' elements such as illness, diagnosis, disclosure, treatment and risk reduction behaviours; nor did we request personal accounts if interviewees spoke generally. Questions about what support was wanted had to be asked carefully as they could be very emotional for interviewees. A final open-ended question about what else people might want was rephrased after the first three interviews, to address what else people might want to talk about – as in the quotation at the beginning of this chapter, from an interview with Ntomboxolo, who had only talked about HIV in support groups and with medical professionals. We wanted interviewees like Ntomboxolo to finish what was often a novel if not stressful experience, feeling that they had said whatever they wanted to – that they were, as she put it, 'satisfied' with their participation in the research.

Interviews were often emotionally intense. Distressing topics such as difficult relationships, parents' bad reactions, illness and death, and the care of children after interviewees' projected deaths were not probed, although many spontaneously discussed them. If people asked medical questions, or requested counselling or other help, we referred them to appropriate services, or asked about the possibility of their using resources to which they already had access – doctors, nurses, counsellors, support groups or family members. Some participants seemed to use the interviews to talk about things in a one-off way that would not have worked if we were going to meet again. Pam, for example, spoke of things she had done that she regretted – having unsafe sex, and having sex with a married man – and that she did not feel able to talk about with her social worker.

The interviews were sometimes difficult for us too. The research assistants had not previously talked with many openly HIV positive people, though they had been involved with HIV awareness courses and campaigns. For me, there were many distressing and anger-provoking moments when interviewees described the absence of MTCT treatment during pregnancy in the late 1990s and the subsequent deaths of infants, or their own inability to obtain treatments that have been shown to be effective – particularly when they were manifestly candidates for ARVs, whose good effects I have seen over the past decade in the British HIV support study.

The project asked participants about their strengths and successes – for instance, in finding treatment, telling people of their status, living 'positively', and in maintaining relationships with their partners at a time when a lot of emphasis had been placed on HIV as a breaker of relationships (Burns, 2002). These were not 'conversational' interviews however. For example, we did not respond as we would to friends when interviewees described their failures to use condoms or their relationship problems, or speculated on their own health and lives. And rather than trying to solve any problems interviewees presented to us, we made referrals to appropriate services.

Where interviews were conducted in Xhosa, the research assistants translated my questions and participants' answers as we were talking. Twenty-nine people were interviewed partly or wholly in Xhosa, eight entirely in English – four of these were men. Female interviewees, though living in similar economic circumstances to the male interviewees, may have had less English-language education, or simply have been less confident about using English. When I returned without research assistants for the later interviews, participants of both sexes who had previously been interviewed in Xhosa spoke in English. It was also clear that participants in many interviews where we used translation understood English well, as they would often respond in Xhosa to questions asked in English.

When co-interviewing, and particularly when translation is involved, there are several conversations going on at the same time. Sometimes interviewees spoke to both of us; occasionally they spoke directly to me in English but on a couple of occasions in Afrikaans or Xhosa, neither of which I understand; sometimes they spoke to the translating co-researcher. Many interviewees were also 'talking' to the broader policy, popular or media audience they envisaged for the research. Mary, for instance, a woman in her thirties, centrally involved in a support group, directly addressed the tape recorder towards the end of her interview, when discussing government and activist campaigns.

A final demographic form and receipt for the interview fee were completed with my and the research assistants' help. Further questions about the research were requested and answered at that point. We encouraged people to return to view, add to, comment on, and, if confidentiality could be maintained, keep transcripts. Everybody wanted transcripts, but few were actually taken away. Finally, we distributed the research fee – cash, as preferred by all the CBOs we talked to in advance, not a T-shirt or other goods, which are often given to research participants in developing-world research. The fee was based on the hourly research assistant rate at the local University of Cape Town. It was, proportionally, in line with the fee given in my UK HIV support research. For the majority of interviewees, who were unemployed, had few working family members and lived in cash-poor neighbourhoods, the fee seemed high. For working- and middle-class interviewees, however, it was a less substantial sum. It was not possible to determine a fee that would be of similar significance to all the interviewees, given South Africa's economically diverse population. Members of one NGO consulted during research planning argued that the fee was too low when disclosure was for many HIV positive people their only income source. We did not, however, want to foster an economy of disclosure that turns HIV into an envied and divisive state. As in many situations of trauma and conflict, journalists were already paying people to 'go public' with their status (Skjelsbaek, 2006). We emphasised that the research fee was a token of appreciation for people's assistance, not payment for an entire life story or for material that would be in the broadcast domain. Several interviewees who worked with community and activist organisations donated the fee. Other interviewees specified the money's concrete value in relation to HIV. Some said they would buy good food. Several described the money as destigmatising and socially including: going home with this money would show their families they were not useless, and could still contribute. At such points, the fee's value in helping draw in diverse participants emerged: these were not the locally powerful people who often become research participants in resource-deprived areas (MacLeod, 2004).

Analysing the material

All words, word fragments and obvious paralinguistic elements such as laughs and coughs in the interviews were transcribed using standard conventions. We included repeated words or syllables, incomplete sentences and minor interviewer interjections such as 'mhm', and anonymised transcripts by proper name removal or substitution. For this book, a clearer text has been created for transcript extracts in the early chapters, where content rather than style is important, and some other identifying information has been changed (Corti *et al.*, 2000). Some textual and semantic clarifications are also included, in regular and curled brackets {}. Transcripts omitted pauses, emphases and other paralinguistic and prosodic features, partly because they are difficult to transcribe reliably without measurement, partly because the scale at which they are meaningful is hard to determine, but mainly because their significance can be variable within and between speech communities, let alone across languages.

'English' interviews were conducted in South African English which differs markedly from British English, and many participants spoke a mixture of English and Xhosa. Xhosa is a historically and socially diverse language, often syntactically complex, sometimes highly traditional and formal-sounding, sometimes full of modern idiom and containing many Xhosalised terms from other languages. Individual and familial idioms also affect people's speech (Bakhtin, 1986). In addition, the interactional context of the research was complicated, involving different participant relationships; co-research, often using translation; and, potentially, a number of different understandings of the research itself. This complexity of languages and interactions made paralanguage, conversational and discourse analyses too speculative to attempt. The research was constrained to concentrate largely on what people said, broad structural features of their talk, and its institutional contexts.

Transcription included, for Xhosa-language interview sections, the research assistants' spoken versions of my contributions in Xhosa and in translation, and the participants' responses, again in Xhosa and English. The quotation at the beginning of this chapter shows this format. A sample of translations were checked by a second research assistant and approximately half the interviewees were given a more detailed language analysis by myself and Lumka Daniel, who looked at word choices in Xhosa and South African English, and lexical equivalence, in relation to common lexicons in these two languages and in UK English. Transcripts were content-analysed, and this material was fed back to the NGOs and CBOs initially consulted about the research. Later, transcripts were analysed for narrative structure. The next chapter presents an overview of themes that emerged from the content analysis (Mostyn, 1985) and forms the basis, alongside the historical and political contexts outlined in the previous chapters, for later chapters' accounts of narrative strategies.

The content analysis evaluated talk about specific support categories arising in each interview as either positive or negative, and noted illustrative examples. This analysis was done by hand because it was conceptually simple, involved a fairly small number of research participants, and the procedure facilitated research assistant involvement. Content analysis did not look at interconnections between categories or interactions between demographic variables and support categories, since participant numbers were judged too small to produce valid data on this.

The importance of particular types of support was judged by the significance interviewees explicitly gave them, and by their frequency of occurrence across research participants. Importance does not, though, map smoothly onto number of mentions, and allocated 'significance' is impossible to scale. For instance, people might talk fairly little about their partners, even when they said they were very significant support sources; and they were unlikely to tell unfamiliar interviewers a lot about the emotional content of those relationships, however strong it was. Often, too, it was difficult to assign 'support' to a particular category when categories overlapped or were too wide. Sometimes these imprecisions were institutionally grounded, as for instance when nurses did counselling, doctors interacted with NGOs and 'family' included the highly distinct subcategories of your own and your spouse's relations. Interviewees' own representations of what was meaningful further conflated the categories. For example, they sometimes made no distinction between nurses and support group facilitators who were 'lay counsellors' with no medical or psychological training; or they made generational rather than relational distinctions between who did and did not support them, between older and younger people rather than biological family members and others. At times, too, interviews provided a lot of material about one form of support, such as relationships with a spouse, or difficulties of disclosure, and then logistically – for instance because the interviewee had to feed a child – stopped. A couple of interviews were shortened because research participants were tired or ill. Interview tapes are also marked by friends or strangers entering interview rooms, noise outside the room, room moves and the activities of children in the room; we treated these not as interruptions but as punctuations of the interviews.

Interviews were heavily structured by the research context. Speaking about a serious health issue, at a time when medical treatment was limited, participants tended to foreground and value medical support. Speaking at a particular political moment of the epidemic, they were sometimes, like Mary talking 'to' the tape recorder, addressing an imaginary audience for the research who might perhaps listen to their demands for better services. Speaking about HIV at all was sometimes very new; several women, like Ntomboxolo, said they had never done this before except with a nurse or doctor or in a support group. Zoleka had told her husband, who, as we saw in the previous chapter, blamed and ignored her. She explicitly compared talking to us to this event:

Zoleka: I am very grateful that I've met people like you with whom I can talk about this thing. Now that I have this thing, I would have spoken to anybody and explained this thing the way I've just done. But even if I would like to, I just feel impatient and discouraged because there are people already that I've told about myself who have reacted badly.

Recently diagnosed interviewees often felt they had little to say; they were still finding out about their health and thinking about HIV's significances for them. Clearly they are going to tell very different kinds of story, with different content, than one of our women interviewees who had talked to the media about her baby's death from HIV-related illnesses in support of the MTCT campaign, and participated in television programmes.

A qualitative content analysis cannot provide a comprehensive or fully reliable picture of interviews. It necessarily will yield a debatable set and weighting of support categories, derived from what are themselves partially expressed views of HIV support. Nevertheless, such work can still be valuable if presented in an open, usable and contestable way (Gibson and Schwartz, 2004), first for the relevant stakeholders – in this case, the NGOs and CBOs initially involved with the research, to whom we took the results from this analysis for discussion. Second, this kind of analysis can demonstrate the importance of high levels of particularity in HIV research, allowing understanding of phenomena that often get ignored in the concern to produce generalisable results. Third – and in contrast to the previous point – a qualitative content analysis of our interviews was also able to demonstrate some commonalities between people's representations of the epidemic in this specific corner of the South African epidemic, and in other contexts of the pandemic.

3 Talking about the big thing

For the past four years, MSF has witnessed first-hand the daily devastation caused by the AIDS epidemic in South Africa and the extraordinary clinical benefits – and hope – that the availability of ARV treatment brings to the community. Our work in Khayelitsha in the Western Cape, where we provide ARV treatment for nearly 350 people with AIDS, clearly demonstrates the feasibility of ARV treatment in resource-poor settings; there is no longer any question that it is possible.

Médecins sans Frontières Open Letter to the South
African government, 12 February 2003, Médecins sans
Frontiéres, 2003

With regard to things that are helpful to one who is living with HIV firstly, you must accept it. When you are told that you have HIV, accept that because that is what will make you live a long life. Secondly, it's good behaviour. If you were drinking and or smoking, you must stop all that. Thirdly, if you are taking medication, you must take your medication as prescribed. Finally, if you have a partner, like, a boyfriend, you must use condom . . . Since I told my family if I'm HIV positive, I'm feeling very well . . . If you go to the support group, there is a lot of things you can get from a support group. If you've got a problem, you can share with other people in the support group . . . If I have side-effects with the tablet or, I'm allergic to one of those trials, they stop me from that trial. So, there is nothing {wrong} because now, I started in 1998, from 1998, 1999, 2000 . . . if I have a problem I can phone Sister {name} and go to {hospital}. If I don't have money I can borrow it from my neighbour and when I come back the sister give R.20 to pay the neighbour back . . . I try to eat good food and even exercise because, every Saturday I go to play a netball. We've got a netball club. So, I'm doing exercise.

Mhiki, Khayelitsha, June 2001

One morning in mid-June, 2001, it's raining heavily. I and my research assistant are splashing across a deserted intersection just outside Cape Town. We dive into our third minibus taxi, the one that will finally take us to the clinic we're headed for. Neither of us have been to the neighbourhood before; I'm from London, my research assistant is from KwaZulu-Natal, now living in Cape Town for the first time to attend university.

The taxi is relatively empty; only people who really have to travel are out in this weather. After waiting around 15 minutes, we take off. The seats are all full now, but the taxi is still luxuriously uncrowded by the usual standards. The driver pulls over and waves his arm in the general direction that he and the other passengers think we should take. With sagging umbrellas blowing across our faces, we trudge down the main track into this section of the township. The ground is waterlogged. Many of the houses, almost all one-room corrugated iron shacks, are developing puddles in their doorways. There will be large-scale flooding in a couple of hours. A man running a small general-goods stall, canopied with plastic, gives us a few minutes' shelter and suggests directions. Finally, we ask the only other person out walking, a woman, who indicates that we should follow her. She takes us on a complicated ten-minute journey between houses, using alleyways and smaller paths, to the door of the clinic. There, amid profuse thank yous, she gives us hugs, and walks back in the opposite direction.

The clinic is freshly painted, and has a once-weekly specialist HIV session, as well as several sessions for TB appointments. It also has the distinct benefit of an energetic and very competent nurse who has set up a peer-facilitated HIV support group, helps members get training in crafts and home care skills, procures food aid and clothing for them, and pushes for their entry into hospital drug trials. But one session a week is too little; sometimes the HIV doctor does not turn up; the TB clinic often will not help people with HIV; the drugs that the clinic is supposed to dispense for HIV-related conditions, thrush in particular, often run out; and there is no antiretroviral treatment, or treatment for HIV positive children in the vicinity.

The people we talk to from the local HIV support group are angry about the situation. Although they appreciate the support they get at the group, the MTCT provision, and the state grants some of them receive, they also want a local HIV doctor, appropriate medicine, a full treatment programme, and more HIV awareness in a slow and bureaucratic grant system that often demands more time and energy than people living with the virus have. They have no money to take buses or taxis to other clinics. If they are ill or looking after small children, they cannot walk there either. These interviewees know a lot about front-line HIV treatments and are keen to use them. They are, as Paul Farmer points out of his Haitian patients, not interested in second-best, developing-world, 'appropriate' care (1999: 21). Unsurprisingly, given their lack of treatment access, they discuss using traditional medicines, but like almost all our interviewees they doubt that they can help much with HIV – and they are very aware that some people are trying to profit from their desperation. This is the research day when the interview fee makes the most difference. In the sudden wet and cold, everyone wants to buy paraffin for their stoves, and very few have the cash for it.

This chapter explores the pragmatic theory that is being constructed within and about the South African HIV epidemic, by people who are themselves living with the realities of that epidemic. It describes our research participants' accounts of their strategies for living with HIV, what they found helpful, and what help they wanted, in the specific circumstances of Western Cape townships between 2001 and 2004. It breaks these accounts up according to the kinds of support that interviewees mentioned, that is, conventional, western medical support; support interviewees provided for themselves; traditional medical support; support from counselling, social services and support groups; family and friendship support; and religious, popular media and political support.

Much of what interviewees said confirmed what other research has found in relation to bonding and bridging social capital (Campbell, 2003; Policy Coordination and Advisory Services, 2006). However, some of what interviewees said went beyond existing findings and policies, generating new suggestions about how to combat the epidemic. These suggestions came pragmatically from 'focus (ing) on what we know works', as Nelson Mandela (2000) advised in his closing speech to the Durban AIDS conference. They were driven by the desire he describes, to move from 'rhetoric to action'.

The account that follows takes participants 'at their word', that is, it deals with *what* they said, not *how* they said it. While some participants gave very clear and vivid accounts, others, less fluent, were as committed to participating in the research, and produced equally important formulations of HIV support. The chapter does not focus on particular individuals, but rather presents quotations from across all the interviews, in order to give a picture of the theoretically and practically important understandings of living with HIV that were developing collectively among research participants at this time.

The chapter begins by considering conventional medical support, because the HIV pandemic is first of all a health crisis, and because medical definitions and treatment of HIV are topics of considerable and continuing debate within South Africa.

Conventional medical support

Most of our research participants emphasised conventional medicine in their accounts of support. Sipho, for example, when asked at the end of his interview if there was anything else he thought would be helpful, simply reiterated his earlier request, 'I just ask for the treatment only.' Some interviews were conducted near clinics, after or before clinic appointments, but the same emphasis appeared in interviews conducted in university and CBO (community-based organisation) offices. This stress on conventional medical support also appears in people's accounts of their HIV positive lives in other situations of treatment shortage or unavailability (Squire, 1999). Even where ARVs have been available long term, this emphasis remains significant. There were, though, wide variations among our South African interviewees in their HIV medical experiences and talk. Men were more likely than women to recount major HIV illness experiences. Women talked less about personal medical issues, for instance STIs and HIV-related symptoms such as genital thrush, although this may have been because they were more likely to be interviewed together.

Medical knowledge

People's knowledge about what HIV is, and about transmission, symptoms, and disease progression and treatment, is central to the debate about ARV treatment readiness. In relation to this relatively new, complex and changing pandemic, knowledge is an important form of support in itself. Detailed and accurate knowledge, though not explicitly investigated in this research, was frequently displayed in the interviews. People were aware of CD4 and, to a lesser extent, viral load measures, even when these were not available to them. Some used weight loss or gain, often expressed precisely in fractions of kilograms, as a parallel or replacement measure of health.[1] At the same time, interviewees did not spend a great deal of time discussing these clinical markers, and placed considerable reliance on personal feelings of illness and wellness. There was also a tendency among symptom-free interviewees to bracket off their HIV status and talk about themselves living 'as if' they were not ill. This strategy, compatible with living healthily and safely, has been noted among people living with HIV in the developed world too (Crossley, 2000; Ezzy, 2000), though it was probably strengthened here by lack of treatment options.

Most interviewees gave accounts of accessing and following HIV and other treatments that attested to their commitment to conventional medical strategies, and their efficacy within medical regimes. Young women's persistence in travelling to a province with MTCT, getting tested and treated, often secretly, and finding plausible non-HIV related reasons for formula feeding were good examples. Many interviewees also described successfully following difficult TB treatment regimes. Others recounted a dedicated pursuit of ARV and other HIV treatments, such as fluconazole for thrush, involving long days of travel they could hardly afford, and constant information-seeking on trials. Monica and Nosisi, for instance, who were interviewed together, attended a local HIV clinic with long queues for the doctor, who came on Fridays only, and medicine shortages. They travelled to another, better-provided clinic about 10km away, but only if they had the cash to do so. The interview fee was going to allow this:

> **Interviewer**: You {Nosisi} had to go to {clinic name}; does anyone else?
> **Monica**: I'm going {clinic name}.

> **Nosisi**: Yes we go there but if you haven't got money you don't take a
> train.
> **Monica**: This is your money now is helping, tomorrow I'm going {clinic
> name}.

In 2001, our few middle-class interviewees, none of whom had health insurance, were in some ways more disadvantaged. Their neighbourhoods had less public HIV treatment, education and activism; they knew less about tests, drugs and trials. Used to relying on the private sector, Pam, for instance, took multivitamins and Bactrim – which acts as a prophylaxis against HIV-related pneumonia – only when her family and friends could afford them. She would not attend a public clinic, lest people recognise her. By 2004, local private doctors like Pam's were referring all patients known or thought to be HIV positive to the public sector, where treatment was freely available.

Interviewees with most experience of HIV services had, unsurprisingly, the most extensive knowledge of HIV treatment. Mhiki, whose story of her successful medical and life regime begins this chapter, had been diagnosed in the mid-1990s when already ill, and enrolled quickly on a hospital ARV trial. She gave a concise account of the regimes and side-effects she had experienced:

> **Mhiki**: I've changed that trial because before I was using AZT, Viread
> {Tenofovir} and others. Now I'm using Zerit {d4T or Stavudine}.
> My trial treatment is good for me . . . the thing about the Viread is
> that I was sick, vomiting and a lot of diarrhoea. So, I stopped it at
> the same time but, the other tablets were good, no side effects.

Unlike Mhiki, most interviewees had had little contact with medical services, but they still demonstrated considerable medical knowledge about HIV treatments. This knowledge came largely from their active pursuit of media information from newspapers, radio, TV and leaflets, and increasingly from support and activist groups.

Evaluations of medical services

Interviewees' evaluations of medical support around HIV differed considerably. Early in the epidemic, many reported having tests with little or no counselling. As we saw in Chapter 1, Michael had avoided thinking about HIV during his first three years of repeated illness and HIV testing in the late 1990s – an avoidance enabled by lack of information from medical services:

> **Michael**: Yah the problem was that I was not even knowing what is it,
> what is this test for. It was just the name of the blood test not
> knowing what it is for etcetera, and even myself I didn't ask . . . I
> didn't get the pre-test counselling and also the post-test.

Inpatient HIV care in the late 1990s, mainly in non-specialist facilities, was often perceived as non-confidential, with nurses writing 'HIV' on files and doors and announcing it loudly on the phone. Such care could also be fatalistic. Monica described getting diagnosed in 1997, while she was in hospital to have her daughter, cloistering herself away from the communal area, with no one to help her after the revelation, and being told directly by medical staff that her daughter would die:

> **Monica**: My food and table is there, and then the doctor is telling me. So after that I'm not going to the dining room again. I'm sleeping, I'm crying. The whole day I'm crying and the Sister is not there now. All those people is gone. I'm only one. I'm crying the whole day and my child that time she is fine and after that when she is one month she is so ill. She is sick. And, the Sister she is telling me that, 'Your daughter is not finish two months, is dying.' They talk like that.

By 2001, HIV test counselling by nurses and social workers was said by most interviewees to be good, focused on accepting HIV, and living a long and healthy life. Other specialist HIV hospital and clinic services were also highly valued.[2] Confidentiality was said to be assured; several interviewees told stories of staff disciplined or sacked for breaching it. Doctors and nurses in HIV specialist settings were valued because they were 'nice', approachable, informative, supportive, friendly and humorous. Interviewees reported they were able to see them as and when they felt it necessary. Of course this perceived change was reported retrospectively, but it seems to indicate some real improvements.

Even in 2001, though, non-specialist clinic staff were described as often rude to HIV positive patients, stigmatising women especially as promiscuous, as other studies have found (Ratele and Schefer, 2002), and neglectful of confidentiality. One interviewee attending a TB clinic when the neighbouring HIV clinic was not open, for instance, said the doctor told her in front of a waiting crowd that she could only be treated on the 'other' (HIV) side.[3] Such disrespect, some interviewees said, could not be reported, as medical staff might lose their jobs. At least in this case, interviewees seemed to regard the possibility of causing unemployment, albeit in a situation of national medical staff shortage, as obviating the right to formal complaint.

Interviewees pointed out some recently improved aspects of treatment itself. Several described being tested in earlier years and not collecting the results. The speed of VCT (voluntary HIV counselling and testing) had had a big effect:

> **Andiswa**: When they said we should get our blood tested {in the antenatal clinic}, I knew. I used to get sick, and then in the clinic they would advise me to get my blood tested and then come at a later date to get the results, so I used to run away and not come back

to collect the results. So on that day at the clinic I thought I was going to do the same thing . . . what happened, they told us not to go home and wait for the results. The results were going to be on the same day, so I was caught. They called me and told me . . .

MTCT programmes were very positively described by interviewees. Counselling, medication, support from nurses, facilitated groups and especially the eventual negative test result for the baby were all mentioned. No interviewees reported a positive test result for their babies – indeed there had been none, at this time, at the clinic attended by most of our interviewees on MTCT programmes.[4] However, confidentiality was difficult to assure. HIV positive mothers had to wait for a bell to sound and then pick up formula from a specific place, practices said to be potentially revealing of HIV status. The cut-off of formula after a child received a negative result was also widely regretted.

Treatment for opportunistic infections and prophylactic, preventative treatment were highly valued, despite being only sporadically available. Interviewees reported that clinics frequently ran out of appropriate medications or operated a triage that seemed irrational. Monica, for instance, criticised the absence of medication that she knew she needed:

Monica: Currently I'm suffering from a throat. It keeps changing sides, becoming better on the one side and starting again on the other side. As I'm speaking with such an unclear voice, it's the throat. There are tablets called (fluconazole) even in this clinic. However, I don't really know what sorts of people get these tablets. From this throat disease I've also suffered from the thrush yet I attend this clinic on a daily basis. I also go to {CBO} at {neighbouring settlement}. It is said that it is the clinic only for people like us who are suffering from this disease yet, I've never been given these (fluconazole) tablets. Yet, when we were with {CBO}, we were told that these (fluconazole) tablets are for the throat, the thrush and the headache but we don't get these tablets.

Some healthier and relatively affluent interviewees travelled to other, better-provided clinics. Some, like Pam, wanted to do this so other people would not recognise them. However, most interviewees thought the value of local HIV-specific treatment outweighed the potential loss of confidentiality, particularly as people are all there for the same reason.

Interviewees all had some knowledge of ARVs. Some interviewees had already been referred to or had found ARV trial or pilot projects for themselves; they evaluated these projects very positively in terms of the drugs' effects and access to support. Mhiki, for instance, having found a drug combination that worked well for her, emphasised the value of also having the phone number of a nurse she could call any time. Two of the male interviewees had just joined a pilot project administering ARVs, with its own support group. In Chapter 1 we heard one of these men, Benjamin, giving an account of his decision-making: a negotiation of medical, political and life realities alongside the frightening stories about side-effects that were current in the contemporary climate of political scepticism and material shortage. The other man was Michael, who felt well, despite a low CD4 count, but was looking forward to feeling better:

> **Michael**: I will see the difference now, I'm already healthy now, I will see the difference, because the main thing is to reduce the virus and stop the infections /mhm/ and just prolong life and live ok.

Other interviewees were strongly conscious of medical facilities' failure to provide ARVs. As Zola said:

> **Zola**: Doctors are treating us as though we are suffering from TB only even though they are also aware of other serious problems like HIV that we have. I don't know why they do that, perhaps it's because there is no treatment for HIV yet. So here in the clinic they have nothing to help us with let alone Panado when you have a cold or fever. Otherwise, if one has some money s/he can go to places that are providing a better service and pay the costs.

Many participants also knew of medical professionals' limitations in this matter, their frustration and low morale (Iliffe, 2006). Nosipho said of her own doctors and nurses:

> **Nosipho**: Yes shame, they are trying in their ways. For instance when we are sick we do not go to the clinic, we go to our special {NGO} clinic on the side. So there, when you are sick they will give you the relevant medication {for opportunistic infections} and multi-vitamins. So their treatment is not enough, because in other clinics they get lots of medicines, those that we do not get here.

At this time, some interviewees did not know that ARVs are only appropriate at a specific medical stage, and thought they should be given to everyone to keep them healthy. Nomthandazo, for example, who was relatively well at this point, wanted ARVs to keep HIV 'at a low level'. In a resource-scarce situation where treatment was perceived as being withheld for political and economic reasons by the government and the developed world, respectively, and where HIV treatment education was not nationally provided, it is not surprising that ARV demands had become overgeneral. When, in response, we asked what people had heard about ARVs and who they could discuss the issues with, interviewees said they could discuss these demands with medical staff and in the support groups they attended, though they had not yet done so. This seemed to be an area where a small amount of information could undo some common resentments about the contemporary treatment situation.

The situation was easier by 2003–4. More HIV clinics were open for longer, but numbers using them had increased dramatically. People still found travel difficult even if – as with city-centre hospitals and clinics with large catchment areas – it was reimbursed. Antiretrovirals and drugs for treating some opportunistic infections remained in short supply, were often out of date, and leakage from the public health system was said to be common.[5]Antiretrovirals were, however, more widely available, and the sample of interviewees that I talked to again had considerable experience of them. Michael was coping with the difficult catch-22 situation of being relatively healthy due to ARVs, but finding fulltime work stressful, tiring and bad for his health. By this time, interviewees not on ARVs, rather than complaining about drugs shortages, tended to say, like Vuyani, 'I don't need those drugs yet'. The national treatment readiness criteria, specifying between 4 and 8 weeks' (Department of Health, 2004) appointment attendance, and preliminary treatment if TB is co-present, was, however, not an easy requirement to meet if you were already ill. Most fatalities in beginning ARV programmes occur in the early treatment period when large numbers of patients enrolled are already severely ill (Médecins sans Frontières, 2003; Médecins sans Frontières, 2004; Médecins sans Frontières and World Health Organisation, 2003). Two interviewees, Monica and Sipho, died during this pre-treatment period.

Non-medical support from medical sources

Interviewees also valued other less strictly medical ways in which conventional medicine supported them, practically, informally and emotionally. By 2004, doctors were key in maintaining grant provision. If ARVs improved CD4 counts, the disability grant would be withdrawn; but health improvements might be transitory, insufficient to allow paid work or, as was potentially the case for Michael, erased by such work. Without the grant, unemployed interviewees did not have money to travel to their clinic or to obtain the good nutrition they knew was required for ARVs' optimal effects. Some doctors were reported to be unwilling to sign disability grant application forms when interviewees perceived themselves as entitled to the grants; most interviewees reported doctors to be more helpful.

Medical professionals were also valued sources of referral to support and training groups. Some interviewees described a time after diagnosis when they could not talk in support groups and nurses or doctors spoke to them individually, gradually encouraging them into support groups. Sometimes nurses ran groups themselves and canvassed resources for them, going considerably beyond their professional remit, as indeed often happens in health crisis situations and with health professionals working in resource-limited situations generally. When Monica and her husband died, the HIV clinic nurse made exhaustive enquiries to locate an uncle who would take in their children, to avoid them going into institutional care. As Zola recognised, it is also outside the remit of the job when a nurse organises left-over bread and egg donations from supermarkets, and obtains old clothes for the support group associated with her clinic.

> **Zola**: {The nurse} help us because she go to ask to these big shops and something and say, 'Come help us with that thing.' But, I haven't got full information but I see is not a thing maybe she supposed to. Is asking for us the old clothes and the old shoes because she think about the group . . . she work for the group, you see.

Medical education about and provision of condoms was also generally valued. As Zoleka said, if the clinic provides these scarce goods, they must be used:

> **Zoleka**: Even my husband, if he doesn't want to use a condom, I tell him to sleep down there on the bed next to my feet on the bed. He mustn't come next to me with his head. This is because I take them there in the clinic . . . . he accepts it.

Doctors were used as sources of information about healthy lifestyle in general, particularly nutrition and exercise, and to provide multivitamins whose most-valued effect was on ability to eat. As Nomthandazo put it, 'The body was weak, rejecting everything so I came to see the doctor, he examined me and saw that I need them you see.' The problematic issue here was that the apparent effects of multivitamins on appetite meant people could not use them if, unlike Nomthandazo, they had insufficient money to buy food. As Linda said, 'These multivitamins make you hungry, they make you want to eat all the time.'

While many interviewees reported using garlic, ginger, chilli and lemon, as recommended by nurses, doctors and indeed the Department of Health, some said these items were culturally unusual enough to be status-revealing:

> **Zola**: If the people see or think about something like garlic they don't understand. They ask me 'What is this thing for?' and then I must explain . . . but, I can't tell my neighbour.

Many participants also reported using the African potato as a food supplement, again following medical and government advice. Its tuberous nature was said by some to be potentially risky, presumably because it might carry soil microorganisms, but the pill form was prohibitively expensive.

A general contradiction emerged – as it often does in people's accounts of HIV-related nutrition – between attempts to eat healthily, and the need to eat calorifically. Some interviewees reported receiving advice to cook without oil and steam their vegetables. Many participants found healthy but low-calorie foods could consume their entire budget. At this time, few interviewees received food supplements or food parcels; those receiving the disability grant reported mostly using it to maintain good nutrition for themselves and their children.[6]

Nutrition and exercise advice from medical sources were often discussed as if they had the efficacy of medical treatments in themselves – a strategy that both indicated a high commitment to formal healthcare, and that was probably a pragmatic necessity in the context of treatment shortage. This strategy did not imply for interviewees the disengagement from conventional HIV treatment expressed in some health ministry discourse on nutrition and exercise.

Finally, interviewees used doctors and nurses as support for psychological, relationship and family issues. Sometimes, they drew on them in unofficial ways considerably beyond their professional remit: as mediators in disclosure, and as counsellors in situations of relationship difficulty. Michael was upset when his girlfriend split up with him, so the clinic nurses called her up to try and arrange a reconciliation. Zola was expecting a nurse to discuss HIV with the woman he was due to marry in a couple of days and who he had not yet told about his status. Busisiwe was trying to lure the girlfriend of her ex-boyfriend to the clinic, so that she could meet the nurse who had previously talked with Busisiwe's mother:

> **Busisiwe**: I found out that this girl who is in love with my boyfriend is also HIV positive. So now she has a this much tall {shows with hand} child. This has made her not want to listen. What happened is that she used to breast-feed her three-year-old child whom I suspect is also HIV positive. So now, I don't know how she feels whether she is still fine or not. I want to trap her and say '{name}, come with me to the clinic, there is a nurse that phoned my mom that I want you to see and simply tell you all those things'. When we get here I would let her hear from the horse's mouth because she wouldn't believe me.

In these interviews, research participants' knowledge of and demand for front-line medical treatment for HIV, their experience of taking responsibility for difficult health conditions in resource-limited situations, and their critical engagement with medical services, suggested that medical support could indeed be successfully extended, for instance, to include ARVs. The interviews thus support the positive findings from ARV pilot programmes referred to in the MSF letter at the beginning of this chapter, and later studies of these successes (Coetzee *et al.*, 2004). We found strong preparedness in a wider group of HIV-affected people for whom ARV treatment was only a hoped-for future. Our interviewees were not just 'treatment ready' in terms of what they knew and whether they attended appointments; they also had a broad, collectively developed understanding of treatment's significance.[7] Interviewees' active pursuit of health indicates, too, that, far from heading towards medicalised dependency on conventional treatments, people with HIV determinedly pursue such treatments, use them effectively, yet still engage critically with them – as, indeed, do people in other developing-world situations of medical resource shortage.

The interviews indicate forms of 'bridging' social capital – links between, for instance, HIV medical staff, NGO and CBO staff, and their patients and clients – as well as 'bonding' social capital – links among people with HIV themselves – that are rarely assessed. They also display relatively high levels of HIV 'cultural capital' (Bourdieu, 1986) – in this case, medical knowledge and wider understandings about HIV and its treatment. Given ongoing low levels of treatment access, and a future of the pandemic that will undoubtedly involve new treatment requirements and possibilities, the development of such capabilities in a resource-constrained area, with little formal HIV education or treatment, has continuing significance for HIV treatment debates in other developing-world contexts.

Self-support

In the interviews, participants frequently described supporting *themselves*. Self-support was not a category we investigated explicitly, but it appeared clearly enough in the material to warrant separate consideration. Often such strategies derived from HIV information or other support people had previously received, sometimes they seemed to develop from non-HIV-related sources – media, religion, politics. In all cases, they were presented as the interviewees' own, actively constructed or endorsed and pursued by them. At the beginning of this chapter, for example, Mhiki formulates her own, complete theory of living with HIV, taking in her whole life. Most interviewees expressed strong commitments to medical treatment, good attitudes and behaviour, stopping or reducing drinking, exercising more – running, football and weights for the men, walking and netball for the women – and healthy eating and drinking, including fresh fruit and vegetables, unrefined foods such as mealie-meal, or corn porridge, and water, juice and bush tea rather than caffeine and alcohol. Zukiswa, for instance, describes a commonly advised drink, presented here as her own:

> **Zukiswa**: I . . . used these carrots, I used cayenne pepper putting it in warm water. Alcohol, I used to drink alcohol and then I paused I was told that I must, er, and then I realised I am someone that has got the virus so I had to drop the pace. Even if I drink, I should drink less, but I gave up, I quit.

Active HIV acceptance was also presented as crucial. Mandisa achieves this by situating illness as a normal part of life, and HIV positive people as normal:

Mandisa: The most important thing is to accept it. So that it can rest as well in your system. And if or when you are sick, you should not always think about HIV even if it is just a headache. Don't think as if you are going to die when you have a headache because of HIV. That will kill you quickly, if you always think about it. You must just accept it. You must think of yourself, not as different to anyone else, you are not different to an HIV negative person, but you must know that you are optimistic.

An internal conversation leading to personal acceptance must occur, constituting the HIV 'self'. Speaking out was also important; silence can kill you, some interviewees asserted. Talking about HIV, to yourself and others, was something that those affected could productively do to help themselves. Telling people about HIV, using themselves as examples, brought interviewees gratitude and fulfilment when their listeners got tested, or began to take their advice on how to live.

These accounts of changes in life may have drawn on concerns about health – around nutrition, exercise, and alcohol and drug use – that were general in research participants' neighbourhoods at this time. Self-help discourses about health issues, partly imported western self-care discourses, partly constructed in South Africa itself, were increasingly current in popular media, but also in policy and everyday talk. Perhaps the salience of HIV strengthened that currency. In western countries, such preoccupations are often criticised as individualising, depoliticising and banalising, fostering managerialism about emotions, relationships and the body (Coward, 1989; Craib, 1994; Lasch, 1991). However, in the South African context of high HIV prevalence and low treatment availability, interviewees' formulations of self-support seemed helpful in building their own effectiveness within medical, psychological and social formulations of HIV. They also pointed towards the use of other 'traditional' and self-medicating forms of healthcare that were, more obviously than conventional medicine, under the interviewees' control.

Traditional medical and self-medication support

Interviewees' engagement with conventional medicine seemed to be supported by their experiences of self-care, using over-the-counter phar-maceutical products such as painkillers, vitamins and antacids, herbal remedies, Chinese and ayurvedic medicines, and remedies obtained by personal appointments with traditional healers. As with conventional medicine, our research participants often relied on media – radio, TV, cata-logues – for information about such treatments. Benjamin was always on the lookout for immune-boosting products:

Benjamin: Like if, I, like I saw a catalogue of medicines and then I find that I do have money to buy that, because I was told that my immune system is low.

Encouraged by powerful brand marketing, a government policy focused on self-care, and perhaps – as with Fana Khaba, the DJ who turned to Africa's solution, or the people who bought Mathias Rath's vitamins – trying to avoid the difficulties and lifelong complications of ARVs, people like Benjamin might come to rely so much on themselves that they do not take advantage of conventional medications as they become available. However, people's skills in managing their own health, worked, our interviews suggested, in exactly the opposite way, giving them expertise in knowing the limits of the self-care sector in relation to conventional medicine. Like all interviewees with access to conventional treatment, Benjamin was concerned not to jeopardise it. When he started ARVs he stopped all other medications. Medical staff did not forbid them, but insisted on knowing what other substances were being taken. They were particularly concerned about traditional medications taken internally, often to produce vomiting or diarrhoea, which they said would upset the stomach and weaken the HIV positive person:

> **Nomthandazo**: They said we must not use traditional medicines you see. You should not vomit, you should not loosen your stomachs, you should not drink medicines that are going to loosen your stomachs. So that is why because if your stomach is loose you become weak.

Traditional and self-care medication are still the primary health resource for 80 per cent of people in Africa (World Health Organisation, 2003). World Health Organisation initiatives this millennium have heightened their profile both as treatments and as focuses of pharmacological research. However, healers are legally bound in South Africa not to offer cures for HIV, cancer and other serious illnesses. Most people do not use traditional healing for serious physical illnesses or contagious conditions when conventional treatment is available. Rather, they access it for small, embarrassing or persistent medical conditions, and sometimes for social and psychological problems. The characteristics of this study – associated with HIV-related NGOs and CBOs, and conducted close to clinics by university researchers – probably discouraged talk about traditional medicine, especially in a local political climate of demand for conventional medical treatments. Traditional medicines produced by healers were also said by several interviewees to be incompatible with Christianity; this ideological conflict may have discouraged others from talking about such medicines. Many of our research participants did, however, regard it as useful and acceptable to apply traditional herbal medications externally for HIV- and non-HIV-related problems, and doctors typically approved this.

No interviewees reported using internally taken traditional medicines for HIV currently though several, like Siphiwe, reported earlier negative experiences: 'I didn't get any help, it just made me mad,' he said. Many interviewees had decided that traditional medications were irrelevant to HIV, as they were to other infectious diseases such as TB. Traditional practitioners were also thought to be financially exploitative in the HIV crisis market. Zola was typical in expressing a general sympathy with traditional medicine but ruling it out in HIV's case, where it served mainly for sangomas – healers who use spiritual as well as herbal remedies – to make money:

> **Zola**: This thing {HIV} is like a job to my people like sangomas and all that. I understand but I don't trust those people but, I believe my traditional but I don't trust sangomas when it comes to this sickness because I find that sangomas have nothing to do with this thing. This is different, that's why I don't think sangomas can take something. I think sangomas can play something with the money to have something to his pocket you see because, I understand this thing is too difficult for sangomas.

Other alternative practitioners were also attempting to extend their market by adding HIV to their repertoire. For instance, Indian herbalists and numerologists operating in the centre of Cape Town, distributed leaflets proclaiming their success with a wide variety of complaints from 'pregnancy problems', sexual issues, 'bewitched people' and promotion difficulties to HIV, indicated by terms such as 'weight loss' or 'night sweats', or simply by the picture of an AIDS ribbon.

Scepticism did not stop some interviewees from hoping that an alternative, affordable, accessible, and preferably traditionally South African treatment or cure would be found. Some discussed, with considerable doubt and caution, cures they had heard about on the radio that claimed to turn you negative. Many ill participants said that they would try such things, if they could get hold of them, since – as they pointed out – nothing else was presently available. As Sipho, very ill, undergoing TB treatment and waiting to start an ARV pilot put it, 'I can {try} because I want to live.' Busisiwe even hoped to find such a cure. She had been taken to a sangoma as her mother had assumed her symptoms indicated her ancestors' call to become a sangoma herself. She was now training, or being 'treated', in order to become a sangoma. However her mother, on discovering her HIV status, was angry at the waste of money; to her, it was obvious that HIV had nothing to do with this calling.

Another ground for HIV's dissociation from sangomas' powers was articulated by Benjamin, whose experience of sangomas countering – and sometimes causing – short-term problems, told him his long-term HIV status was something different:

> **Benjamin**: I was still working there and there, so they {family} keep on saying, 'maybe there is, this is not something like, a, witchcraft?', I mean, you know, we Xhosas as we, we, like if someone is, jealousy of you is gonna go to a sangoma, 'I don't want that guy to be promoted from the work he must stay where he is', something like

that. I told them 'no I've been in the witchcraft for time ago, time again but this is from the doctor, not now, long time ago'.

After 2001, easier access to ARVs decreased interviewees' talk about traditional cures. However, many participants spoke of trying doctor-approved substances alongside ARVs in a kind of ongoing experiment:

> **Nosipho**: I want to, like use the medication that I get from the clinic in conjunction with traditional or Xhosa herbs and then monitor the progress.

Subsequent clinic-based interview studies, asking more direct questions, have reported high rates of complementary medicines' use, alongside ARVs, in South Africa, as in Africa and the US (World Health Organisation, 2003).

Interviewees who did not reject traditional medicine because of religion or commitment to conventional medicine, found traditional and self-prescribed medicines to be valuable, with external herbal preparations and non-prescription medicines from pharmacies being the most accepted. They wanted to use these substances in conjunction with conventional medicine and in consultation with doctors. They planned to research and spend money on them – when they had it – as part of their active pursuance of health, and alongside their own regimes of nutrition, exercise and psychological self-care. This approach exemplifies the holism endorsed by many progressive conventional and traditional medical practitioners in developed and developing worlds. Many interviewees were, in addition, aiming for the state of physical, mental and spiritual balance that characterises traditional medical notions of 'health' (Mkhise, 2004). However, their approach to self-care also operated as a pragmatic negotiation of possibilities within the epidemic.

Even before increased access to ARVs, then, our research participants were articulating a dialogic engagement with health knowledges and practices. Such engagement has been characterised by Rose and Novas (2004) as a claim to 'biological' citizenship. The 'self' may be constituted as 'biological' by regulatory authorities such as medical institutions and government, but the 'subjects' of these authorities can also negotiate, on the grounds of their 'vital rights as citizens'.

Counselling

Interviewees usually described counselling in connection with the HIV antibody test. Since it was often provided by medical professionals, it was not a clearly distinguished support category. For instance, Mary did not call her supportive exchanges with her doctor before the test, and for a year, 'counselling':

> **Mary**: I did not get any counselling. I only heard that my child at {hospital} has HIV. One of the doctors came to tell me why the child

was sick. But before he told me, he asked me if I had any information about HIV. I told him a little bit, just what I used to pick up from radio and TV. He then asked me a question as to how I would feel if my child was sick because of HIV. I told him I would accept it. He then told me yes, it was HIV. He also asked me how was I feeling then. I told him, I had accepted it. However, after he had gone I was left alone with several questions in mind. I was wondering how I was going to explain the matter to my parents and my boyfriend. I didn't tell anyone for the whole year. It was a secret between the doctor and me only.

Interviewees rarely mentioned counselling by name without being asked about it. For most, it seemed to be less significant than the longer periods of support offered by clinic staff, support groups and family.[9] Sometimes, too, interviewees said it had not happened as mandated. Nevertheless, interviewees' descriptions of it suggest that despite its institutional and linguistic unfamiliarity, it had considerable though specific value. As with members of TASO, the Ugandan HIV support organisation (Kaleeba *et al.*, 1997), participants here said that counsellors had promoted a positive, life-affirming acceptance of their status, had diverted them from negative and suicidal thoughts, and had been helpful in dealing with distress after the result:

> **Phumla**: There was, yes, encouraging us as well. S/he said when I was leaving, people should not see me. Like, you must not show it people that there is something, like it should not be obvious to people. Relax, get out and they must not see, really. I got out relaxed.

But one-off counselling could not magic acceptance into being for Phumla, or for others like Nosisi:

> **Nosisi**: The counselling was difficult. I was crying. I wanted to just die . . . the counsellor was helping . . . she was counselling one time but it's just shocking because you cry.

Some interviewees were aware that they could return for subsequent sessions; a few had taken up the offer. Lindi for instance came back the same day:

> **Lindi**: I was shocked when I was told and I could not listen, I went out. So that lady {counsellor} followed me, but I did not pay attention, I left, I took a taxi, I went home. And then when I got home, I realised I might have missed something by not listening to that lady, so I went back again.

Most research participants, though, said that they had only needed one counselling session as they had 'accepted' their status. As we have seen, some planned to ask or had asked nurses to counsel family members. Some women whose children had died of HIV-related illnesses returned to counselling, usually for one or two sessions, often with the same person who provided post-test counselling.

One-to-one counselling thus seemed useful to our interviewees only in emotional crisis. They did not relate it much to other potential HIV counselling goals – behavioural risk reduction, disclosure and relationship advice.[10] They understood it in a quite specific way, as an encouraging intervention at a crisis moment, that did not provide practical help. The 'acceptance' it promoted was not full acceptance but a *determination* to accept, the beginning of exploring HIV identities and practices, to be continued in family and support group discussions. This beginning was nevertheless often described as a transformative moment.

People make similarly episodic use of counselling services in developed-world epidemics. African-origin clients in these epidemics are particularly likely to be seen as underusing counselling services (Elliot, 2006). Such underuse may result from counselling's fixed-term form and its lack of social engagement. In the Ugandan organisation, TASO, family involvement is indeed encouraged after initial one-on-one meetings (Kaleeba *et al.*, 1997). People may also want 'therapeutic' help with HIV from other services – for instance, social work (Gilbert and Wright, 2002). In this research, interviewees said that what they called 'counselling' should be close to the educational outreach that nurses, rather than counsellors, did within families and communities, and to what support groups achieved. Nosipho, for example, said:

> **Nosipho**: I wish there could be people to teach to people so that they can understand and accept it because the people with the virus are also human and they can live longer . . . I wish there could be counsellors who can explain to people what's going on so that people can learn to understand what HIV is. Because once someone is found to have HIV, it's not HIV but it's AIDS to people.

Interviewees such as Nosipho, who were in support groups, were often performing in this way as 'counsellors' themselves.

Support groups

Support groups, hosted by public clinics, NGOs or churches, were valued positively by everyone with experience of them. Most research participants did not have full family support, and almost all wanted to be involved with support groups.[11]

In the context of HIV's stigmatised and gendered character, the specific nature of support groups was significant. Some women preferred women-only groups on the grounds of confidentiality:

> **Nosizwe**: Men won't fit in. No they won't fit it because sometimes you are not ready to talk about your issue and then your neighbour would be here. Men no, it's like they would talk about it. It is better for nursing mothers and other women who don't have children, that would not be a problem. Men no.

Some men thought it was easier for men to talk in all-male groups, although groups for heterosexual men had – as in other HIV epidemics – been difficult to set up. Our male participants' involvement with groups was lower on average, and they seemed more reliant on partner support. Benjamin, for instance, had for four years talked only to his girlfriend about his diagnosis. During that time, she got tested and became a regular attender at support groups, and, performing the gatekeeping role women are assumed to take in family health, eventually induced Benjamin too to access HIV services. Several women interviewees were similarly planning to get their male partners in touch with support groups.

The few interviewees with experience of mixed groups liked them, and said women and men were able to correct misconceptions about each other. The pattern of developed-world HIV support groups moving from integrated to more specialised provision during epidemics seemed, therefore, in this high-prevalence context, to be reversed. Those with little experience of HIV services thought gender-specific provision was necessary. Those who had been in mixed groups suggested that HIV 'community' usefully crosses gender lines. However, consistently fewer men attended gender-mixed groups throughout our study. Such groups seemed to be sustained primarily through women's activity. Perhaps this was because the groups involved not just informational, socioemotional and practical support around HIV, but 'female-identified' activities such as talk about relationships and children, food distribution and cooking, clothes distribution, and small-scale craft income-generation projects, in all of which men participated less.

Group size and childcare provision at support groups were not – as they are in developed-world settings – treated as significant issues. People were too concerned with having a group to care much about size, and women were used to having small children with them in clinics and social settings. For many interviewees, transport costs prohibited attendance at any but their nearest groups. Some healthier interviewees used the walk to a group site and back as exercise. A few chose more distanced groups because of greater anonymity, groups' specific political or training remit, or particular facilitators. There was some disagreement over whether facilitators were necessary. The majority who discussed this topic thought they were, mainly to initiate on-topic discussions. As Tandiswa put it:

> **Tandiswa**: We wouldn't start if s/he {facilitator} hadn't arrived, we would just chat whilst waiting for the milk {formula}. It's only after s/he had arrived that we would start.

Facilitator gender was not discussed, but facilitators were valued for being warm and maternal; one was praised for hugging group members and seating new or quiet members by her. Facilitator HIV status was not perceived as significant, as it often is in the developed world. Even positive participant status was important mainly to ensure confidentiality. Family members would also be welcome in groups. Many interviewees considered them conjoined by their HIV concerns rather than seropositivity, and frequently said HIV-affected relatives also needed support.

Groups set up within MTCT and ARV programmes have specific member-ships, educational aims and monitoring functions. However, it seemed these groups discussed whatever issues their members wanted, and interviewees expressed strong ownership of them. Many such interviewees also had experience of more general support groups, and reports of how these groups worked did not differ much.

People cited a variety of benefits from support groups. They were a good source of information – Sipho, not yet in a group, said group members seemed to know everything. Indeed, participants' experience of groups seemed proportionate to their knowledge of HIV issues – the more they reported attending, the more they knew. Groups disseminated advice on HIV-related illnesses and treatments, and on nutrition and exercise advice. Frequently, members exchanged information about their own symptoms:

> **Nosisi**: It help us because we share. She can say 'eh, I've got a thrush' and then me I can say 'I've got a gusto' and, she go to say 'how you help your gusto' . . . Then I say, 'the doctor gave me this and this or, tell me when I've got a gusto I must take that charcoal and then I'm going to be alright.' Since we share, since me, I was going to the group, I'm feeling alright. If I didn't go to the group I'm going mad because that thing is in me. I can't sit with the other people because I didn't go to the group.

Perhaps the most generally cited gain from groups, as this quotation also demonstrates, was socioemotional. Realising that you are not alone, and that there are others like you who are managing to live open, healthy and happy lives, was inspirational for many interviewees.[12] As Nomthandazo, diag-nosed during her pregnancy and part of an MTCT support group when we interviewed her, put it:

> **Nomthandazo**: When I got here {group} I was still in shock but then they explained that every one of us came to fetch the milk formula and we are all the same, that is when I got free.

The groups made participants feel they were the 'same' as others and they had rights. Group discussions reduced stress, made people stronger by encouragement, and enabled disclosure – Nomthandazo, for instance, said her experiences in the groups led her to 'tell out' at home.

Such support is not 'help' in the commonest, practical sense, and interviewees often noted its purely communicative aspects:

> **Interviewer**: What is helpful there {in the group}?
> **Zukiswa**: It's talking only. You get it out, that it's like this and this. Every person that comes in we tell them, we don't hide from them. Even if it's someone we know, maybe someone from next door would show up you see. You have to then start talking because she is here for the same reason that you are here.

As this description indicates, confidentiality is assured when you are all attending for the same reason. If someone says she saw you there, she is disclosing herself by saying this.

Groups supported – but did not force – formula feeding, condom use and disclosure. Interviewees, especially those newly diagnosed, seemed to use the groups to formulate strategies around these practical and social issues, as they used counselling to move towards personal belief and acceptance. How to disclose, and to whom, were rehearsed at length. The history of silence in the South African epidemic, the emphasis within test counselling on the benefits of disclosing when you can, and perhaps also the recently implemented guideline of disclosure to one person in order to access ARV treatment, meant that speaking out had at this point assumed powerful individual and national significance.

Groups were often described as being like families – as has been found in other post-trauma situations (Mukamana and Collins, 2006). Recently diagnosed people often spoke of the groups as their only support and saw no end to their attendance. This caused concern to staff in MTCT programmes which aimed to induct women into family and community-based support networks by the programmes' end. However, even the women most attached to their MTCT groups were actively planning to tell family members about their status. A year on, most were rarely seen by the facilitators. Interviewees who were longer-diagnosed had mostly already disclosed their status to family members, with generally positive results, and some had made friends from support groups whom they saw outside. The two interviewees with the most experience of support groups said that for them, the groups had outlived their usefulness for coming to terms with HIV positive status. They found the groups' new-diagnosis preoccupations somewhat annoying – something that characterises longer-diagnosed people's reactions to such groups in developed-world epidemics also (Squire, 1999). Two long-diagnosed interviewees beginning ARV treatment were, however, finding the group set up specifically to support that treatment useful. It may be that, in future, as in some 'older' HIV epidemics, groups for newly diagnosed people can usefully run alongside other specialised groups, for instance, for people beginning ARVs or dealing with their long-term use and effects (Jelsma *et al.*, 2005), and training and income-generating groups.

Negative aspects of the groups, for instance the difficulty of seeing very ill people, were not often mentioned, though the shock of seeing people dying from HIV-related conditions was remarked in other contexts. Perhaps because of the stigmatisation of HIV's visual signs, as well as practical transport difficulties, relatively few clearly ill people attended the groups. Some groups' exhortatory style was not liked; a few participants mentioned feeling out of place among louder, more confident support group members. Criticisms may have been inhibited in our study because many interviewees received notification of the study from NGO or CBO support group facilitators, which may have made the research seem connected to the groups, despite what we said about it.

Support groups' focus on practical help increased during the years of the research. Food, as well as talk, was always important. Interviewees suggested various combinations of hot drinks and cold food that could be provided without disrupting the groups or inviting interest from other people using the same building. They wanted food parcel distribution, particularly at groups for mothers. They also wanted more skill-building and income-generating activities, and this became more and more of a priority as they adapted to positive lives:

> **Mandisa**: We would like to do something. We would like to do handwork, like sewing, beads, knitting, we would like to do such things.
> **Amanda**: Any job I can do, I don't have a problem, I can do any job.

Group members with access to training and income-generation group projects valued them and would travel to them, even if they were only modestly renumerative. As in TASO's Ugandan work, which emphasises income generation, such projects had limited potential in the current economy and interviewees recognised this. However, training and income-generation groups did operate for some as entry points, often through volunteering, into paid work as counsellors, home carers, and advocates for pregnant HIV positive women, thus demonstrating elements of 'bridging' in addition to their powerful 'bonding' social capital. HIV service requirements are large in high-prevalence contexts such as South Africa. Support groups are important mediating institutions between HIV positive people, as patients and as themselves providers of HIV services, acting to reinscribe them as social and economic citizens.

The South Africa notion of *ubuntu*, a rather inexact description of which would be 'common humanity', extends 'family' beyond biology to both the local and universal human community (Sigogo and Tso Modipa, 2004). Support groups were in this study the social formation that most often approximated this ideal. However, while they were the highest-valued forms of support for our research participants after medical care and family, they were, as we have seen, not a fixed resource. Their nature varied as people progressed from diagnosis and MTCT programmes, to longer-term issues of how to survive economically and how to use drug regimes to keep healthy. South African HIV services do now include more groups specifically for men, groups for those on ARVs, and groups providing training or craft opportunities.

Some of support groups' most important effects – promoting acceptance, optimism and community – could be fulfilled in other settings. In Uganda, day centres for HIV positive people are described as helping people feel they are not alone (Kaleeba *et al.*, 1997). Here, interviewees sometimes constructed their own informal support groups. Several women reported establishing supportive friendships with other women from their groups. If support groups were not running, some people built up friendship networks within clinics. Vuyani, for instance, was in the habit of meeting other HIV positive people at the clinic and getting advice from them on how to live; these informal contacts let him know he was not alone:

> **Vuyani**: Like here I found out that there are many people like me, understand. So I do not keep this thing in my heart.

Family and social networks

Support from family

The interviews showed that, as one might expect, families and friends were major supports for people living with the virus. Disclosure seemed to lead, as in other contexts, to more social support and less depression (Schmidt and Goggin, 2006). Most participants had had good reactions from family members, especially sisters and mothers. Sylvia's description of her sister, for instance, recovering from initial shock to give Sylvia hope about living with HIV, to urge her not to worry, and to promise confidentiality, was characteristic:

> **Sylvia**: She was only told by me of my HIV status on the third day {after leaving hospital}. No I told her, 'Sisi {sister}, what they found out there, they said I am HIV positive.' She was shocked, but in her shock she tried to make me feel strong. She said, 'In whatever you do, don't even keep this thing in your mind.' She said, 'People like that do live with this. You need to take this thing easy, and not keep it in your mind.' She said, 'I will also try, I will keep it a secret, I won't tell anyone.'

Time since diagnosis, as well as contact with support sources such as nurses, counsellors or groups, seemed the main factors related to actual and planned status disclosure.[13] Benjamin, having disclosed only to his partner for four years, told other family members once he himself started to attend a support group. Interviewees in MTCT groups who had not yet disclosed were all aiming to do so – often, if their babies tested negative after nine months, or when they next saw parents living in rural areas, or simply when they were 'ready'.

Family members were usually reported as saying they felt the same about the interviewees as before. Often their response was immediately to accept what could not be changed – very much the 'acceptance' experience interviewees reported of themselves. As Tandiswa said of her mother, 'she accepted it, because it had already happened'.

Relationship success after HIV disclosure was high among our research participants, and was related by them to a variety of factors: trust; length of relationship and the children in it; having a close 'me and you against the world' relationship; talking about things; love; shared religious faith; and not blaming each other:

> **Vuyani**: My wife . . . was found to be like this as well . . . So she said, when she came to tell me, she said 'eish you would have to accept this, I found out that I have this in my blood'. I then said 'yah there is not problem because this is not your fault and then we are still going to live'.

Interviewees not currently in relationships mostly said future partners could be of any HIV status, though a few were looking for HIV positive partners. Michael, for instance, wanted a strong HIV positive girlfriend so that the two could support each other. A few female interviewees had decided, after their diagnosis, never to have another heterosexual relationship. As Ntomboxolo put it:

> **Ntomboxolo**: I don't want to see any other man sister, sorry about that. In my lifetime, I cannot be involved in a relationship. I have learnt my lesson, that they are not good it's obvious.

At the time we did the study, interviewees' HIV positive children were generally very young – or had died – whereas most interviewees were still healthy. Disclosure to children was usually done or planned for when children were around 12, but was also related to the severity of parents' illness, as other studies (Armistead *et al.*, 2001) have found. Younger children were said to show signs of being relieved by the information, again as has been found in other HIV epidemics (Murphy *et al.*, 2001).

Late-teenage children had more trouble accepting parents' diagnoses. Benjamin talked about his status to his whole family and to other young people he knew, but found his own daughter very resistant:

> **Benjamin**: I must educate them {young people} because they are in love, they got affairs outside, they come at night and leave at night.

They come when the morning comes . . . I wish to speak to them, so that they must know what is wrong what is right and how people you know, mostly used to be infected by HIV, and I'm also having a child who's sixteen years old. So by talking to my nieces, I know they gonna talk to my child, you see, like when I talk to my daughter, sometimes she doesn't want to listen to me.

As in other crisis situations, interviewees' responsibilities to their children were driving their survival. They were striving to stay alive to ensure their children's future. Pam, for instance, wanted to save enough money to provide for her daughter's tertiary education before she died; others with more short-term hopes were arranging their children's care after their death (Mukamana and Collins, 2006). Their children's deaths, and their own deaths as parents, were some of the most difficult issues for participants to talk about, and the research did not pursue them. For one participant, Monica, the issue of childcare was, as we saw in Chapter 2, still not fully resolved at the time of their death.

Where relationship breakups were associated with HIV, it was generally through partners' difficulties in dealing with implications for their own status. For example, Tandiswa's partner was emphatic that he had nothing to do with it and that she 'brought it'. When interviewees' status was known more widely, this affected how partners would be perceived, as with Michael's former girlfriend, with whom the nurses tried to effect a reconciliation, but who could not cope when his status became widely known. Three interviewees mentioned relationships that had ended primarily due to their status. Nosisi described rather briefly and fragmentarily, at different places in the interview, her own relationship breakdown, within the context of her generalised belief that HIV destroys marriages:

Nosisi: Me I was married, and had to leave it . . . My brother {co-interviewee} was right when he said it breaks down a marriage because I was also married.

Some interviewees had experienced hostility within their families. Benjamin described his family's reaction of seeming to accept his diagnosis, but then giving him his own crockery – a reaction his determined education of them had now undone. Busisiwe gave an account of continuous difficulties, of a kind experienced by many women interviewees. She had an HIV positive child; her HIV status thus had large implications for her mother's own life as a mother, grandmother and carer. Her mother had a son, also thought to be HIV positive. She now 'feared all her children would die of this'. She was, too, as we have heard, furious to have paid money to a sangoma when her daughter's problem was not an unheeded spiritual calling, but an illness associated with promiscuity: 'My mother say "wu my God you have the HIV positive, wu wu wu! I waste my money for {traditional} doctor", you see.' She repeatedly pointed out the stigma of having an HIV positive, sexually transgressive person in the house:

> **Busisiwe**: My mum embarrasses me with that {HIV} even in front of people because I'm HIV positive. It makes me feel not at home, as if I'm lost. It makes me want to stay outside. Even when I've made a minor mistake like spilling sugar, she would say, 'This is because you are thinking of guys and AIDS and all that.'

Monica described another characteristic failure of family disclosure – where it leads to the breakdown of the confidentiality that, for instance, Sylvia's sister had assured:

> **Monica**: I told {name} my brother's wife because I don't have a mother or grandmother or anybody. So, we tell all our issues to an older person. She insulted me and exposed the issue all over the township. One day we were in conflict she insulted me saying, 'piss off, this thing that has AIDS'. At that time I had not told even my husband. I also got into conflict with my husband. He was asking what {name} was talking about when she said I had AIDS. I told him she was just insulting me.

Problems also arose with family members who needed support themselves to deal with interviewees' status. Many were said to be very sad, others excessively anxious about interviewees' minor illness, and others again, to deny the diagnosis by refusing to talk about it. Mhiki's sister was 'worried' when she told about her status: so 'now, I try to give her counselling and support, and she is fine now'.

Support from friends

Many fewer people had told friends than family about their status, mostly, it seemed, because apparently non-HIV involved friends were judged less likely to maintain confidentiality and were considered more distant than family members. Those who had told apparently non-HIV-involved friends included three out of seven male HIV and only two out of 27 female HIV positive interviewees. These disclosures had not affected friendships. Their HIV status had been, interviewees said, forgotten in the relationships, although they still talked openly about HIV and encouraged their friends to get tested. As is said of non-HIV affected friends in other HIV research (Squire, 1999), people were not receiving support from these friends so much as giving it, and in our interviewees' cases they valued making this contribution.

The generally negative valuing of non-HIV positive friends by the interviewees did not hold true where, in Busisiwe's case, there had been limited family support:

> **Busisiwe**: I go to my friends and to the elders and say, 'I have this problem, what words do you have as advice?. Then, when s/he speaks s/he would say, 'I believe you should go for the treatment because the medical treatment and pills are good.'

An important aspect of this reported response was that it focused not on socioemotional or informational support, but on treatment. Busisiwe was describing her post-diagnosis situation in a rural area where treatment possibilities were minimal, but clearly known about. The support Busisiwe reported also contradicts common suppositions that rural areas with few HIV services will be the most difficult and unsupportive places to disclose.[14] It may be that our participants' majority situation of living in relatively new informal settlements, with few family members around them, alongside people from many areas of the country – and increasingly, from outside the country – with considerable population mobility as well as high unemployment and crime, made friendship and community support less likely and 'bonding' social capital lower than in more established urban or rural settlements. Perhaps these factors led them to value family support more highly in consequence.

People's representations of neighbourhood responses were usually extremely cautious. Monica was one of the most positive when suggesting that:

> **Monica**: with regard to the township it differs. Some people don't want people with HIV and others they are very helpful to them.

Monica had, however, had to move away from one area because of her status:

> **Monica**: I became uncomfortable with the people of {township name} because they were complaining that we were using their toilets yet we had AIDS.

Several interviewees made generalisations about the 'people' of the country which suggested support from local communities generally was limited. Zola asserted that:

> **Zola**: Some people get shocked if I tell them of my HIV status because we, in this country are anticipating that one who says s/he has HIV should have sores, be dirty and that's how we know it . . . Even your neighbour would put whatever s/he has on paper because you are disgusting to her/him since you have HIV.

Support in the neighbourhood and from friends, which we could again describe in terms of *ubuntu*, was, then, not commonly described. Nevertheless, after medical care, support groups and family, HIV-involved friends were the most important support resource. Such friends were often made in support groups or clinics. Women from the MTCT groups, telling others they had met at antenatal appointments, visited each other outside:

> **Zukiswa**: That is why my heart is not aching because (of) . . . my time to be with my friends to chat chat chat and these women I know from here {support group}, I visit them during the day, and we will sit and chat about this.

Since men participated less in support groups, they had less access to such HIV friendship resources. Even those that did have them, seemed to have maintained their pre-diagnosis friendship networks more than women, perhaps indicating the greater stigmatisation women face. Certainly, women's disclosure patterns to friends and family differ from men's in other areas of the pandemic (Kimberley *et al.*, 1995).

Disbelief

Many spouses, family members and friends were reported as refusing to believe participants' diagnosis initially, a refusal that was particularly likely when the interviewee appeared well. People knew in theory that HIV did not itself make you look ill but they still expected warning signs such as the 'sores' Zola mentioned, thinness and exhaustion:

> **Benjamin**: My aunt and the rest of the family they believe me. But they worried, but what makes them to disbelieve me again is that is nothing I mean wrong with me I'm still active.

Another reason for disbelief was that people who talked about having HIV were thought unlikely, because of its stigmatised character, actually to have it.

> **David**: Most people do not believe me. Guys, I mean it's not a problem, it's up to them /why?/ Because I am talking about it. Some people I mean most people don't talk about this virus. When someone has this virus, doesn't want to talk so I think they find it strange for a person who talks about it.

Some interviewees were even thought to be misrepresenting their status with an eye to the financial rewards available to those who disclosed in the popular media. However, HIV stigma could also be argued to make disclosure *more* likely to be true; for what payment could possibly erase it? Benjamin, who had disclosed his status to a journalist, found his friend convinced by this: 'He says, "I believe you, you would not just be doing this for money."'

Finally, since some saw HIV as a retribution for sexual transgression, disclosure might not be believed if the person was monogamous – particularly if their more sexually active friend or relative was HIV negative, as in Mhiki's case:

> **Mhiki**: My sister was sick {upset} because she say to me now, 'I don't know if it is a real thing because you never sleep around. You were good lady. It's only me', because my sister was sleeping that side and that side and that side.

Disbelief was particularly frequent in partners, perhaps because interviewees usually told spouses first, in order to safeguard their spouse's and other sexual partners' health. This has been found in other national contexts (Greene and Faulkner, 2002). Such information had far-reaching implications for spouses' and their children's health and lives, making it even harder to assimilate. Women were more likely to have encountered disbelief as they generally tested before their partners, because of pregnancy or an ill child. As Linda, who discovered her status through an MTCT programme, described it:

> **Linda**: My husband, the one I am married to, I told him. At first, he could not accept it, he gave me too many problems. I then continued talking about it every day, I used to chat about it so that it would sink into him that I am HIV positive. Truly, eventually he accepted it.

Disbelief in earlier days of the epidemic could be paralysing, as in Michael's case. By 2001, when HIV's significance and extent was widely appreciated, it could be an opportunity to educate, to reinforce your knowledge and understanding by conveying information to others, as Linda reported:

Disclosure

Research participants often described disclosure to family members as being necessary for health and social reasons. It was also presented this way in test counselling, and in clinic guidelines on ARV regimes. As Nomazwe summarised it:

> **Nomazwe**: {My sister } is the one . . . if I get sick at least there should be someone that knows.

In addition, disclosing helped expand the family support available:

> **Mhiki**: I was worried about my child before I told my family because my sister is taking the child to {hospital}, I don't want her to open

my daughter's folder. So now I'm happy. I don't care no matter whatever. She took my child to {hospital}, I don't care because she knows she is HIV positive. And even now if I'm sick, they know now what is happening.

Representations of disclosure often went way beyond such instrumental criteria, suggesting it produced an internal mental and emotional calm that also led to physical health. Far more frequently than in the UK, interviewees connected worry or stress to physical ill health, and presented the link as medically validated:

> **Amanda**: {Doctors} talk to us, they say one should not keep things within, one should find someone to confide in, a person must find a person to share with because once you keep it to yourself you will lose weight, so it's better to say the things that you don't like so that it gets out of your system.

While such representations are common in popular psychological accounts of mind and body across the world, in South Africa they also exemplify the traditional healing principle of aiming for physical, social and spiritual balance with the environment. In Benjamin's account, keeping HIV 'inside' you like a poisonous secret, and yourself hidden away 'inside' too, will kill you. Getting it, and yourself, out into the open space of disclosure is not a cure, but it is an important element of treatment. This concern to get people into the HIV 'open', though guided by politics and conventional medical knowledge, fits with a traditionally homeostatic account of the world:

> **Benjamin**: You'll find that this guy is, he likes to sit alone, he likes some darker rooms whereby there will be no one who gonna disturb him and, what do we know about a person who acts like that he's killing himself without I mean taking a knife or a gun by sitting alone he just killing himself. . . . So like when I visit people like that I like to make an example of myself . . . I started to make friendship with them by coming with my medical records and show them, 'look this is the tablets that I'm using /mhm/ . . . I've been in and out in the hospital according to appointments, I was sick just like you but I never gave up /mhm/ I never let myself sleep the whole day . . . But you, sitting here you don't want light in your room, you don't want anyone to, within two years we are going to bury you. But if ever you can come out and join us, we won't think about burying you for, within two years we'll think about that later. You'll reach six years to seven years because you gonna learn a lot outside'.

All interviewees reported current or past concerns about family and friends' stigmatising reactions which affected disclosure. Those who had not told partners or other family members, sometimes expected them to react badly because the relationship was already difficult or finished. They feared also that confidentiality would not be maintained. Nomthandazo for instance knew that telling her husband could lead to insults from his family:

> **Nomthandazo**: My husband's family, we are not close you see. So if I tell him, maybe one day we will have a fight and he'll talk it out and then it won't be nice you see. So I can't tell him. I'm sorry I can't.

Other possible serious disclosure consequences were abuse, and the withdrawal of economic support. After testing positive, Andiswa, as we saw in Chapter 1, had moved to her sister's crowded house so that she would not have to negotiate status-disclosing condom use with her boyfriend. Andiswa's reason for not telling her sister was also common: the lack of support available for her sister, of the kind from which Andiswa had benefited.

> **Andiswa**: It's worse for her because she won't have a support group to attend, nothing will support her. She will sit down and watch here at home. I would be going up and down, and she will be thinking that 'this child has HIV'.

Interviewees had extensive criteria for assessing how people might react to their HIV status: listening to their comments about radio or TV items on HIV and on family members or friends known or suspected to be HIV positive; raising the topic for discussion; evaluating the information's likely effects on recipients' health. Illnesses such as diabetes, blood pressure and heart conditions, particularly of mothers, were frequently cited reasons for not disclosing. The difficulty of telling mothers, especially something that will cause great distress, was frequently described (see also Skjelsbaek, 2006; Squire, 1998).

An increasingly significant factor was direct family experience of people getting ill or dying from HIV-related conditions. Some interviewees reported these experiences as enabling disclosure. For others, such as Busisiwe, the existing weight of HIV illness and bereavement made disclosure harder. Religious beliefs were also mentioned as an indicator of likely reactions, as were personality characteristics. People you could not disclose to were often described as being 'funny', a term with many connotations in both English and its Xhosalised version, including maliciousness, being gossipy and drinking too much.[15]

Non-disclosure also caused difficulties, as with Nomthandazo's continuing distress about the husband she could not tell. Where interviewees had not told their friends about their HIV status, they said they felt less close to them, especially when issues around HIV came up. For women on the MTCT programmes, the demands of a young baby meant they saw their friends less than before. However, many said they now had no friends except those made through HIV support services, because they could not be open with former friends. Nosipho encapsulated this position:

> **Nosipho**: None of my friends know that I have HIV . . . our friendship is still the same. The other thing is that since I got a baby I don't have friends any more, not those same friends. Like now the friends I have are the people that I attend the support group with.

Non-disclosing acceptance

Even without disclosure, HIV was often implicitly addressed in friendship groups as members were increasingly affected. A culture of non-disclosing acceptance seemed to be developing among many women, who told each other they had to use formula because they had breast infections, for instance, and often talked *about* HIV together without disclosing their own status. Many interviewees said that despite not disclosing, they tried to get their friends to change their attitudes, as they had. Busisiwe, for example, wanted to use 'Homeless', a song about being an outcast, by Ladysmith Black Mambazo, to do this:

> **Busisiwe**: What I want to do though I'm still with the women's association, is to kind of concentrate on the youth as if I'm joking. There is a song about sleeping in the caves. I'm going to make an example with it as to what it means to sleep in the caves, what causes that especially, when you are still young for example being HIV positive. I will also tell them about other diseases like TB as to what happens when you do not treat them. I have accepted this and in the place where we stay, the youth doesn't want to come to the clinic even though the disease is widespread in that part of the area.

As we have seen, support-giving was viewed as a support for participants themselves. But it was difficult to give support while concealing HIV positivity, as it usually generated questions about the speaker's own status. Desires to give support functioned in the interviews as a plan, but also as a kind of future ideal: a picture of how interviewees would operate, fully disclosing and open, if they were not constrained by stigmatising families, hostile communities and their own vulnerable parents and children.

Non-disclosing acceptance was more problematic in sexual relationships. Several interviewees reported having partners who they suspected were HIV positive for various reasons: partners' detailed knowledge of the topic; illness or death of partners' previous girl or boyfriends; medication partners were taking; or their acceptance of interviewees' own HIV status. At times, women and men saw each other taking multivitamins and eating healthily, and silently surmised positive status:

> **Pam**: He {boyfriend} doesn't know {my status} but we use condom or sometimes we don't use it. mhm/ I don't know I didn't ask him but er, I'm suspecting something, he's HIV that one /mhm/ although he did, he doesn't want to tell me. Like me, I don't want him, I'm also suffering from this virus /mhm/ and he's also but he don't share to me /How, what makes you think that?/ Because I saw some tablets I saw Cozole {antibiotic}, multivitamin /right/ in his drawer and the big tablets, like Lucozade, very big, for energy.

Such assumptions could be dangerous. Several times in this interview it emerged that Pam did not always use condoms with partners although she thought she should. Once, for instance, she and her possibly-positive boyfriend had sex without a condom because:

> **Pam**: I was drunk /mhm/ (laughs) /yeah/ anyway, I didn't mind I go for it /mhm/ because I do love him and he loves me.

This kind of decision-making is common among HIV positive people across the world. In this case, however, the partners' HIV statuses were not disclosed, and Pam was herself ambiguous about what happened; she wanted, in general, to use condoms.

As is apparent from the quotation, and the levels of hesitation and repetition in the transcription, some aspects of sexuality were difficult to discuss and we did not pursue them further since the interviews were relatively short and one-off.

In the field of family and friendship support, interviewees debated the relative merits of 'need-to-know' disclosure, disclosure as promoting physical and mental health, disclosure required by health authorities, and disclosure that is politically endorsed or economically renumerative. These debates were at least as complex as similar contemporary debates within western contexts (Greene and Faulkner, 2002). In addition, *non-disclosing* acceptance, while having clear limitations, was in some cases operating as a provisional means of support. While non-disclosing acceptance seemed to have been largely superseded in the areas where we were researching, it remains widespread across the country.

What can be discerned overall in interviewees' accounts of their relations with family and friends is a highly diverse pattern of support that is perhaps more positive than might be expected. In 2001, these relationships were in the process of becoming an HIV support 'community', albeit an uneven one. Interviewees were remaking existing relationships and making new ones, producing networks of associations and succour that could include HIV as a condition of everyone's lives.

Faith

Religious faith appeared central to most participants' lives and was spontaneously mentioned by many. Even those who said they did not attend church, described spirituality as an important resource. Except for members of one support group, who received food parcels from a pastor, no one reported material support from churches. Such practical functions of religious institutions have, however, expanded in South Africa since the beginning of the research.

One of the most significant forms of religious support related to funerals, which must be well attended to provide social commemoration:

> **Mary**: It's fine to go to churches, but to my church we don't talk about this, I don't know to {about} others . . . On Sundays the weather is fine for me because when you dies, you need them to come – it's for that {that you go to church}.

One interviewee had told her pastor of her status. Another had left her name in a folded paper on the altar, among those of others with 'incurable diseases' who were prayed for at a specific, quiet time. Other interviewees were members of churches which prayed for HIV positive people generally; these interviewees often said they would like to disclose to other members.

Prayer was sometimes conflated with claims of cure – something about which interviewees expressed ambiguity, occasionally wondering, since no other remedy was available, whether there might be something in it. Hoping for such miracles, of course, is understandable in this situation of medical underprovision.[16] Nosipho, the least doubtful of all our interviewees about cure claims, said she wanted to 'confess' to her pastor and try for such a cure:

> **Nosipho**: If you endure to {keep going to} {church name}, they say you get cured. Like you tell the pastor you have this problem of HIV. He says he takes that away. When you come back for a blood test, you won't have HIV, if you endure to going to church non-stop.

Such speculations did not occur in the 2003–4 followup interviews, when treatment was more widely available. Even in 2001, Nosipho herself gave many reasons why she could not always get to church; she was happy with her support group, did not think about HIV too much and accepted her condition.

At this time, most participants simply thought prayer could help you when sick, giving you physical as well as mental strength:

> **Mandisa**: It is helpful because if you are sick you need to go to church so that some things don't catch you that easy . . . It is helpful because sometimes I would be disturbed then go to church. I get there and

that thing would go away. I would rejoice in church and talk to
people.

One interviewee thought religious faith had enabled her parents to accept
her; Sipho credited it with sustaining his marriage. Vuyani also thought faith
had brought acceptance for him and his wife:

> **Vuyani**: I think it is because I go to church, like if maybe I was some-
> body else, maybe I would not have accepted it.

. . . and he thanked God for his HIV negative child.

Some interviewees described religion's main benefit as a kind of 'spiritual
boost' gained from worship and from being, at church, the same normal,
happy and believing person they had been before:

> **Ntomboxolo**: Oh, it helps me a lot. I love church so much. It is where I
> spend most of my time . . . I am a very nice person in church. I do
> not worry. I just live my normal life and no one knows {about} me
> in church.

Maintaining identifications outside HIV is reported as important by many
HIV positive people, and for Ntomboxolo and others, religious institutions
allowed this. Yet the effects of discriminatory or neglectful religious
discourse about HIV are not thereby entirely negated.

Interviewees' religious explanations of HIV were divided. Some, like
Benjamin, saw HIV itself as a direct mark of people's transgressions: 'Church
cannot cure, it is the devil's work.' In this case, God can help you overcome
it. As Vuyani put it, 'it is the devil that does these things . . . it is God who is
going to solve the problem'.

Other interviewees viewed HIV as divine retribution visited collectively
on the ungodly world. Pam, for instance, saw HIV as punishment for a
society with high rates of adultery, child abuse and incest:

> **Pam**: I'll say it's a punishment from God /mhm/ there are unclean things
> that are happening in our country. So God has just put this virus to,
> *isibetho*.

Pam's final word, in Xhosa, means 'sacrifice', like those made by David
in the Bible to keep the plague from Israel, and that of Isaac prepared for by
his father, Abraham. Pam had, indeed, lost an HIV positive child. 'Isibetho'
is also the word used to describe the troubles mentioned in Isaiah (53) when
people are wounded or afflicted for others as well as their own wrongdoings,
as in Pam's account of HIV. In such accounts, the epidemic and its solutions
are all God's work, as many religious accounts of other crises, conflicts and
genocides suggest.[17]

In both forms of explanation, healthy living is devout living. As Pam argued, God will help if you believe; medicines have to be taken with prayer. The mere existence of biblical accounts of calamitous epidemics seemed to provide an assurance that HIV could be lived through. Vuyani was one of several who remarked that:

> **Vuyani**: The bible talks about these things, that in the years to come there will be incurable diseases, you understand.[18]

Vuyani thus frames HIV within an overarching faith narrative. He thinks God will overcome and 'rebuke' it, but he does not think that belief leads directly to cure.

Few interviewees talked explicitly about traditional belief systems in relation to HIV. Busisiwe, however, reported dreams in which she had seen her ancestors holding up sangomas' beads in the shape of AIDS ribbons, to show that everything was alright. Others mentioned believing in their 'culture' in a general way, viewing such belief as compatible with Christianity. For many South African Christians, particularly those belonging to evangelical denominations, belief in ancestral spirits is fundamentally non-Christian. Interviewees' evangelical Christianity sometimes came into conflict with traditional approaches to illness, because of these approaches' links to ancestor beliefs. However, as Mkhise points out (2004), indigenous spiritualities conceptualise ancestral spirits as intermediaries between human and divine worlds, thus making them compatible with at least some versions of Christianity. Most interviewees had a pragmatic approach to the different conceptual frames involved with conventional medicine, traditional medicine, Christianity and traditional faiths. As Busisiwe put it, referring to the clinic, traditional beliefs and Christianity, 'I must take care of it {HIV} on three fronts including church' – and she asked God to allow her to find a cure, to which she would be directed by her ancestors. Such coexistences of belief have a long history unlikely to be broken by contemporary challenges from evangelism.

Religious institutions have played a mixed role in the South African epidemic, as they have in other national contexts. Pathologising accounts of HIV date largely to earlier years of the epidemic. Today, the Catholic Church provides antiretroviral drugs and strongly debates condom use. Moslem organisations accept HIV positive members and do extensive charity work around the epidemic. Major Christian religious figures such as Archbishop Desmond Tutu and his successor, Archbishop Njongonkulu Ndungane, have foregrounded HIV in their discourse, and call for condom use and antiretroviral treatment. Most traditional healers understand HIV as illness, not spiritual transgression. Equally as important for our interviewees were individual, accepting pastors, who led supportive worship communities of largely non-disclosing HIV acceptance. The interviews suggested the value of churches' practical involvement, and of a general spiritual support that does not focus on cure by prayer. Faith also provided vocabularies and forms of ethical discourse that, as we shall see in Chapter 5, could be drawn on to discuss HIV.

Social services

We stopped asking about social service support after pilot discussions because it was so limited in extent. Some research participants mentioned social workers helping with children – which is indeed predominantly how they are deployed within the epidemic – providing HIV counselling, and giving advice on nutrition and sexuality. Pam, for instance, had a social worker because of her HIV positive child, and had received such advice. She could not, however, speak to the social worker about condom use, because she believed she would be told 'I must strictly use a condom, safer sex'. This she did not always feel able to do. She was, as we have seen, willing to be flexible about using them. She also found cutting out alcohol, as the social worker advised, very hard:

> **Pam**: The social worker told me I must stop drinking . . . because alcohol also suppressing your immune system more especially, brandy, but how can I, I'm a socialite, it's very difficult.

Other interviewees wanted help from social workers for caring for positive children, and for telling children about their parents' HIV status.

Non-governmental and community-based organisations

NGOs and CBOs were mentioned very favourably by research participants as medical information and treatment providers. International NGOs were not subjected to analyses, like those made by the government, of their neo-colonial agendas for self-interest. Local organisations were not taken to task for their lack of accountability or self-interest. Given the contemporary resource shortage, such criticisms might seem unlikely. Government negligence, and the discriminatory practices of medical professionals, family members, friends and employers, were, however, thoroughly dissected, suggesting the NGO sector was performing well by comparison. Activist and educational organisations were frequently mentioned, and were sources of strength and inspiration to many interviewees. Participants reporting such involvement tended to display good medical knowledge around HIV and to have disclosed successfully to many family members. Although these characteristics could be precipitators, not results, of organisational involvement, participants' own accounts, and the under-resourcing of public sector HIV education and treatment up to 2001, suggest the latter. Interviewees also approved of NGOs' and CBOs' associated support groups, in particular the additional income-generation activities in which people participated after or alongside the groups:

Nosisi: This {activist} movement helped me clear my mind because if you go there you see and hear everything. Yet at first the movement called {counselling organisation} also found me. It took me under its banner and showed me that I was not going to die, that this was not the end of life. I was not going to die of the disease that I had. I had to do things with my own hands. So now I know how to do bangles and ribbons. {Counselling organisation} showed me that this was not the end of life.

Popular media

Very few interviewees – two – had access to information via the internet. Relatively few reported printed information sources as being important; those who mentioned newspapers usually accessed them second hand, often at the workplace. One support group was using a US-produced advice book-let on healthy living with HIV. As we saw earlier, they read it thoroughly but sceptically, particularly owing to the price of its recommendations and its incommensurability with their lifestyles. Several interviewees mentioned using radio – probably the major HIV information source across the continent (Iliffe, 2006). From it they found out about the virus and medical treatments, but also about exercise, nutrition and non-prescription treatment of opportunistic infections such as thrush, for which there was poor access to conventional treatment. Zukiswa took notes about such radio items, 'If they say what helped someone I write that down'.

Hearing other people with HIV talking on the radio about living healthily, disclosure and having relationships, was also encouraging. Vuyani credited radio with making him aware of the virus 'when this thing was new to people, people did not bother'. More explicit questioning might, I think, have produced fuller accounts of extensive radio use.

Television items about HIV were also remarked on as helpful. *Soul City* was the only media product specified by our interviewees, despite the high profile of other media 'brands' such as loveLife. They generally had television access to *Soul City*, though they also mentioned its radio and magazine outputs. For some, visual media were too much to deal with, too emotionally intense, especially soon after diagnosis. Public figures who disclosed their own or family members' HIV status in any media were viewed as important models. However, popular media could also be the source of worrying stories about antiretrovirals' side-effects, or sensational tales of cures. These messages produced mixed responses of hope, disbelief, suspicion of the makers' profit motives and frustration at their own inability to access or afford them. The conversation of Miranda, unable to access treatment for opportunistic infections, and Mhiki, using a successful though sometimes difficult ARV regime, about a recently radio-broadcast claim of cure, exemplifes this ambivalence:

Miranda: We only hear from the radio, no one has tried but, we do believe because we want to try but we must get something first, money so that we can buy it.

. . .

Mhiki: Sometimes I was excited before. But now, I decide to leave because people lie to us because they want our money. They say they can make you to be HIV negative. So, I don't want to use any traditional {thing} even if I hear it from the radio or, whatever because people want to grab our money.

Politics

At times, interviewees spoke specifically about the local, national and international politics of HIV support. They generally chose to discuss government policy, which they defined as positive insofar as it involved MTCT programmes, and negative insofar as it restricted medications, and failed to provide a state system of funeral funds – a common contemporary complaint in South Africa, frequently made also, for instance, by pensioners' groups. Nor did government help people thrown out of their homes because of their HIV status – a very frequent fear, and a reality for two interviewees. People making negative assessments often suggested that the government was too affluent to care about poor HIV positive people. One woman whose baby died at the time government was resisting MTCT programmes wondered, indeed, whether anyone in government had HIV at all. The government was also said to set criteria for disability grants that required people to be close to death. Mhiki, taking antiretrovirals in 2001, exemplified a frustration that has since become commoner, and that was voiced by other interviewees using ARVs in 2003–4:

Mhiki: I think there is a problem between HIV positive people and the government because the government does not want to give the disability grant. They want to wait until you can die before they give you the grant, and, it's a problem as you can't have food. It's a problem. I don't know what to say to the government to {get them to} give us the money. Because I can't go to work. I've got two kids and I'm on and off {health-wise}.

Women from MTCT programmes had a greater appreciation of government. For example, they were willing to credit the government with other treatment initiatives, particularly in the light of the government's legal fight against pharmaceutical companies' patent restrictions. Such political goodwill was very notable in a discussion between two friends, Nosipho and Amanda:

Amanda: . . . because AZT was recently introduced, those pills that you take when you are 8 months pregnant. They came from the government. It is the government that supports them. They are very supportive as far as I'm concerned.

Nosipho: Like they give us hope with the pills they are trying to get from other countries you see. They give us hope that we are still going to live. Maybe there will be hope that it can be cured.

Amanda: And they say if maybe they find medicine or pills, the prices will be affordable even to the unemployed with HIV, they can afford to buy them and use them.

Most interviewees also discussed how the economic and infrastructural problems of their lives impinged on the epidemic. Nosisi gave a typical general account of this kind:

Nosisi: A person who has HIV does not die of HIV rather of poverty ... Another thing, if you are a sick person, you must stay in a clean environment unlike in a place like mine in (a) shack. The place is full of water and the living conditions are appalling.

In a country with as strong a history of political awareness as South Africa, we might have asked more about participants' perceptions of political support. Even without such questioning, though, a structural 'political' analysis of HIV support emerged spontaneously in almost all interviews. Interviewees produced thorough analyses of their economic, employment and housing requirements, for which they needed 'support'. They described economic shortfalls, which did not let them buy medical care, good housing or food, as their fundamental 'support' failure. Asked to picture how support could be improved, many said they just needed a job – any job – or training. However, many also reported that their employment abilities were limited by their condition. For this reason, income-generating support groups, based locally and involving flexible and physically less demanding forms of work, and other HIV-related work such as home care and counselling, were viewed with enthusiasm.

Participants' responses pointed to complex understandings of the political contexts of HIV, and to their own commitment to effecting change through paid and voluntary work, and campaigning within and outside their neighbourhoods. These capabilities have already driven many neighbourhood responses to the epidemic, through voluntary service provision and activism, but they could perhaps be called on, more generally than they are, in formulating local HIV policies.

Female participants' responses, particularly concerning group support and their development of wider HIV networks, suggested that women living with HIV in this, as in other situations in the pandemic,[19] are often the leaders in developing support strategies that work, for themselves, their communities and for HIV 'communities' more widely – something to which gendered perspectives on HIV and 'development' are increasingly attuned.

Conclusions

Some recurring themes appear in the interviews. Research participants tell of the value of support groups, especially for women without other support, and just after diagnosis. They describe relatively accepting family members, partners with whom relationships can usually be sustained, old friends who do not know, and new HIV friendship networks. Alongside feared, as well as experienced, stigmatisation, they indicate a level of 'bonding' social capital, relations of trust and support in families and HIV-affected groups and neighbourhoods, perhaps underestimated in more behaviourally focused research.

Interviewees also present a very clear picture of their medical knowledge and demands around HIV. They emphasise the importance of religious feelings, if not institutions, for their wellbeing, of media engagement and of cultural representations, particularly those that are open and accepting about HIV, such as public personal disclosure stories. They present a complex political picture of lives lived with HIV in a resource-poor context, structures of local support, and their own actions to enhance these structures. These factors suggest high levels of knowledge-based cultural capital, and of 'bridging' social capital – links connecting people's local HIV organisations with others outside the neighbourhood, often at larger levels. Again, conventional assessments of people's strategies for living with HIV tend not to recognise such forms of capital.

The interviews raised a number of issues that support organisations involved with the research and working with HIV generally in South Africa were encountering in 2001, and are often still encountering, and that appear in other developing-world epidemics: the integration of conventional and traditional medical knowledges, the importance of peer support and activist groups, familial and gendered patterns of support, and the role of faith.

The interviews also demonstrate research participants' pragmatic effectiveness in dealing with the contemporary everyday realities of HIV, while still working towards improved conditions for living with the virus. Interviewees' pursuit of conventional medical treatment; their parallel uses of alternative treatments; their creative development of support communities; and their ability to articulate their HIV experiences within a larger picture of themselves and the world, all exhibit this pragmatic HIV citizenship. Such an approach also characterises the responses of successful HIV organisations in South Africa. It also resembles effective community responses to HIV epidemics described in other developing-world situations (Farmer, 1999).

The content-based account given here leaves out some important aspects of interviewees' responses. As the last section on political support indicates, interviewees often addressed areas beyond HIV. Their accounts of their lives frequently positioned them, not as 'HIV positive' people, but as people 'just like' others – much as is seen in accounts of living with HIV in other contexts (Squire, 1999). Some issues, such as sexuality, the death of children and one's own future death, were hard to talk about. People's talk about 'acceptance' also sounded ambiguous, counterposed to their descriptions of the shock of diagnosis.

The partiality and incompleteness of this chapter's analysis of the interviews comes about both because the analysis imposes support categories on people's often quite general representations of their lives with HIV, and because it takes a realist approach to those representations as more or less accurate accounts of realities. In this case, such realism might seem justifiable. The crisis of non-representation in the South African epidemic, as well as the practical effects of HIV speech – through, for instance, disclosure, campaigning, medical information or misinformation transmission – suggest that it is reasonable to assume the significance of talk about HIV, and some relation with action. However, there were aspects of interviewees' representations that a content analysis could not deal with. One important aspect seemed to be the stories interviewees told, their structuring and how they were told to the researchers, and to co-interviewees. The following chapters look at the styles of narrative representation that participants used.

4 From othering to owning

Speaking out about HIV

it gets awful lonely
lonely;
like screaming,
screaming lonely;
screaming down dream alley
screaming of blues, like none can hear
but you hear me clear and loud
echoing loud;
like it's for you I scream

> from Bloke Modisane, 'lonely',
> in Moore and Beier, 1963: 210–11

One of the themes that has emerged repeatedly is the tendency, even among those who are most concerned about the problem, to portray HIV/AIDS as somebody else's problem. People almost overwhelmingly put the locus of change beyond their own constituencies.

> Cathy Campbell, 2003: 191

When you get to the support group you introduce yourself and confess that you have the virus, you don't hide it. They might ask you, 'How did you feel when you were first told?', so you might say that 'I felt like somebody else', maybe another person might have been worried, the other cried, the other one would have been hard on herself, do you understand? We get there and talk about these things, especially when it's just the familiar faces without the new beginners. We will sit and chat and have fun.

> Ntomboxolo, June 2001, Khayelitsha

Stories of living with HIV

January 2004. I am on holiday in a mountainous area of the Eastern Cape. HIV prevalence in the province stands at 28 per cent; treatment is not commonly available, though an NGO ARV programme started two months ago, some 70km away by road (Department of Health, 2005a; Mtathi, 2005).

I ask one of the workers with the community-based holiday company, what happens to people in this area who have HIV. He says there are not many HIV positive people here. Those that have the virus, contracted it in the cities. People in his village, he says, abstain from sex before marriage, and this protects them. I ask what happens to people who do have HIV, and he says they are cared for and taken to local clinics and hospitals, where there are, he knows, appropriate medications. The nearest tarred road is a couple of hours' walk, and the local clinic is 10km away, so this is a time- and money-consuming activity. A young man, injured in a fight that night, has to wait all the next day to get a lift to hospital. In the meantime, a sangoma, or healer, makes a herbal dressing for the wound. There may be many reasons for not wanting to talk much about HIV, especially when a tourist is asking. HIV is said not to be here much, and not to belong here. But it is also said to be cared for and treatable.

April 2004. I'm visiting a friend who works in a hospital near Cape Town, in a township where HIV prevalence is over 25 per cent among reproductive-age adults (Department of Health, 2005a). A man who is picking up some neighbours from the hospital offers to give me a lift afterwards to a nearby taxi stand – we will all be making a contribution towards the petrol. The man opens the car door for a thin woman who has been sitting on the ground, her head on her knees. It is a warm day, but she is swaddled in sweaters, coughing, her face shiny with sweat. Her sister carefully helps her in and we drive them to another hospital where she is to be admitted. No one asks them for petrol money. As the woman walks very slowly towards the entrance, supported on her sister's encircling arm, the driver watches in silence, and then says tentatively and with concern, 'I think that lady may have HIV', and we agree that she might.

By 2004, many people in South Africa not directly affected by HIV understood and accepted it, in both rural and urban areas. The generality of HIV's effects, and the availability of some treatment, had brought about greater openness. Even in 2001, most of our interviewees had been able to disclose to someone; some had told the whole neighbourhood. By 2004, public figures were talking openly about their own and family members' HIV. This state of affairs seems to indicate a change from 1998, when Gugu Dlamini was killed after declaring her positive status. Yet even at the end of 2003, Lorna Mlofana, an HIV activist like Dlamini, was, like her, killed when she disclosed. People living in high-prevalence rural areas might still, like the man described at the beginning of this chapter, represent HIV as a small-scale issue affecting others elsewhere. This chapter looks at the uneven and incomplete moves from othering to owning the virus that have occurred within South Africa over the past ten years. Chapter 1 examined this shift through changes in policy and treatment; this chapter addresses it through stories told by people living with HIV.

Silence about, stigmatising or 'othering' HIV were common political and personal responses to it in the South African epidemic's early years (Joffe, 1997). This chapter charts moves from 'othering' towards 'owning' the virus, in the double sense of declaring that you have it, and taking charge of it, in our interviewees' stories of HIV support. The chapter argues that these complex and detailed stories make up 'theories' of how change can happen in the South African epidemic. It explores the shape and significance of the stories, as well as elements of HIV experience that are difficult or impossible to represent within them.

As the previous chapter showed, looking at *what* people say about HIV support, treating their interviews as research resources (Plummer, 2001: 36ff.), raises salient issues, in particular around the topics of medical knowledge and effectivity, disclosure experiences, and support from families and friends, religious faith, and the media. However, a content-oriented approach does not consider *how* people talk about HIV.

Although interviewees were asked about HIV support, rather than their own lives, they often responded by telling personal stories: both narratives of specific events, and more general accounts, following the temporal and causal sequences of their lives.[2] Several interviewees declared explicitly that they were going to tell what they called 'my story'. Michael, for instance, when asked about his experiences and expectations of HIV support, told a complex narrative of his life with HIV which lasted around half an hour. It started like this:

> **Michael**: Firstly, eh, sh, should I start my story from '97 /is that where you want to start?/ yah I mean I started to know my status, started to, I mean started to know in '97.

Similarly, David began the interview with a continuous, though much shorter story, of his life with HIV:

> **David**: My story I think it will be very short because er I've just known myself that I'm HIV positive just last month.

To ignore such stories, to refuse to see them as topics of research in themselves (Plummer, 2001: 36ff.) would be to fail the material, and the people who made it available to us deliberately, and with considerable personal effort. Of course, many participants had told similar stories to their families, to doctors, in support groups – and to themselves. Nevertheless, telling such stories seemed an important part of people's engagement with the research.

Many of the stories told of people's moves from 'othering' HIV, or ignoring it, to being open about it and 'owning' it. These stories seemed to be important means both of representing changes in HIV lives, and of bringing HIV itself into representation.

Telling HIV stories

We have seen in Chapter 2 how significant the social contexts of the interviews were for *doing* the research. These contexts needed to carry equal weight in *analysing* the stories the research participants told. 'Context' is a rather imprecise word for the discourses – the social, cultural and political structures of meaning and power – operating across the interviews (Foucault, 1979; Parker, 1998). The research considered interviewees' stories as performed within a set of interconnecting discourses. Narrative is itself a kind of discourse: a form of language invested with particular historical and social significance. At the same time, the research was interested in new theoretical possibilities created within the stories, through the discursive reformulations they performed.

This 'contextual', discursive approach recognises that in performing narratives, we draw on cultural resources, histories and social formations, being 'storied' by them at the same time as being active and effective story-tellers (Labov, 1997; Mishler, 1986; Plummer, 2001: 44; Ricoeur, 1984; Riessman, 1993). It also recognises the importance of storytelling as a mode of communicating social, cultural and ethical structures in many national contexts, particularly in Africa (MacIntyre, 1984; Mkhise, 2004).

Representation is a more complicated process than the mirroring of reality assumed in the previous chapter. It is particularly significant, indeed 'epidemic' (Treichler, 1988), around stigmatised conditions like HIV. The epidemic is often discussed in South Africa through popular representations, rather than directly. HIV is itself freighted with concerns about death and sexualities that popular media throughout the world address repeatedly and intensely. Popular representations are clearly significant for people living with HIV themselves. Many South African interviewees – as in the UK – spontaneously discussed popular media representations of HIV, even though they were not asked about them. Which TV personalities and politicians might be HIV positive, and who had come out publicly about HIV positive family members, were central, not peripheral, matters for discussion, intimately tied up with their own lives. It would be surprising if cultural representations did not affect *how* people living with the virus spoke about HIV, as well as *what* they spoke about.

The synergy between everyday and cultural representation is, as we have seen, the focus of many significant South African HIV initiatives such as the *Soul City* and loveLife campaigns. This chapter and those to follow look at that synergy from the side of the audience, not the cultural producer. The chapters are interested in a broader range of representational resources than those found in popular media, in particular, story genres found in social, religious and political contexts – the full 'symbolic content' (Campbell *et al.*, 2005) of HIV. They work on the assumption that people's relationship to representational resources is an active and creative one, within which they critically and pragmatically deploy and remake representational forms, constructing theories about HIV within the interviews, and within their own lives.

Research on personal HIV stories generally ignores cultural patterns of HIV representation, or interprets them only as contributing to the pathologising victimisation of HIV positive people. Often, though, the cultural form of people's personal stories about HIV are highly significant.[3] The forms on which this and the next two chapters focus, are those of *genres* (Todorov, 1990) that include specific plots, characters and themes. Genres are not historically or culturally fixed, and some are more powerful than others, but they all belong to cultural discourses of storytelling. An individual story can also belong to more than one genre. Stories told about HIV may then be told within a number of personal and popular representational genres, all of which will be relevant to their meanings and effects. Such stories may, too, generate new genres from older ones. Because genres have cultural currency, because they offer narrative 'progression' through events and because they are flexible, evolving to respond to new situations, the genres within HIV stories can also operate as a form of local theory, explaining particular events, usually those that are not yet well known or understood.[4]

It seemed to me that, as in other HIV epidemics, a number of genres were being deployed in South Africa to tell HIV stories. 'Coming out' stories have proved useful models for personal HIV narratives in the west (Patton, 1991, 9–10; Squire, 1999). In popular culture, western HIV narratives have often taken a form closer to horror or the Gothic (Williamson, 1989). In South Africa, HIV stories seemed to be told in ways that connected strongly with common forms of cultural representation, but were also affected by a general trend towards intimate disclosure stories, focusing consistently on 'speaking out' as a route to 'owning' HIV.

As we saw in the previous chapter, interviewees' accounts of their own and others' disclosure and non-disclosure were frequent, detailed and complex. Sometimes, the stories sounded like those told on US and South African television talk shows, radio soap operas and magazine problem pages. At other times, they resembled self-disclosing talk within, for instance, religious and political discourses. In what Kenneth Plummer calls 'intimate disclosure stories', personal, often stigmatised identities or events concerned with suffering (1995: 50) are 'told out', as Nomthandazo put it, in a public arena, leading to redemption or transformation. Plummer suggests that such narratives have a common form. They move from imagining the issue, through articulating it, towards specifying identities, formulating social communities of support and, lastly, setting up a culture of 'public problems' (1995: 126). Intimate disclosure narratives must be told within what Plummer calls 'interpretive communities' of listeners who can, at a particular place and time, 'hear' them, as people 'heard' about HIV in the two anecdotes that begin this chapter. In these circumstances, the stories can became part of new cultural repertoires, which may in turn have wider cultural and political effects. Plummer (1995: 22; 2003) delineates a history of such narratives across the last 100 years in the west as a kind of 'democratisation of personhood' through personal narratives, resulting in a fourth realm of individualised, representational and materially effective 'intimate citizenship' (1995: 146, 151).[5] Examples include slave narratives, African–American autobiography, women's autobiographies (including stories of rape, sexual abuse, domestic violence, feminist consciousness raising), coming out stories and illness narratives including those around AIDS.[6] We could also include autobiographies under colonialism, working-class autobiographies and the process of HIV's 'internalisation' in other African countries like Uganda (Iliffe, 2006: 129). The consequences of the *absence* of such heard and effective stories in the HIV pandemic were well summarised in ACT UP's Silence=Death slogan.

The intimate disclosure genre can operate as a useful 'theory' of the new and hard-to-understand condition of HIV. Its clear temporality lets it articulate causality. Its highly 'personal' nature gives particularity to phenomena that have been over-generally understood. Its cultural currency affords it commonality.[7] Perhaps then, there is a partial, contingent and pragmatic truth attached to intimate disclosure stories, within their specific discursive contexts.[8] This chapter examines the intimate disclosure genre in our participants' interviews, to elicit its strategic value in the South African epidemic.

Intimate disclosure narratives of acceptance and openness about HIV seemed crucial for our research participants. The alternative, a silencing failure to accept, has, indeed, many problematic consequences, at individual, social, cultural and national levels. It can lead to failure to get tested and diagnosed; the minimising of HIV as an illness and failure to seek – or provide – treatment. It may also support social stigmatisation and prejudice, expressed in the failure to acknowledge HIV as a condition affecting oneself, or its displacement onto other people or types of people, other conditions such as TB, or other undeniably important problems such as unemployment, poor health or racism. Perhaps there can be some silent, non-narrated acceptance and 'ownership' of HIV. As we saw in the previous chapter, some interviewees described a non-disclosing acceptance of the condition. But it seems such subtleties must exist within a broader context of open HIV citizenship in order to work. For HIV acceptance is never just an individual psychological state, but always one that is socially modelled and mediated. It needs to be owned and communicated at many levels if it is to be effective.

From othering to owning

It is often remarked that HIV in South Africa has been not just neglected but actively silenced, 'othered', and positioned elsewhere, even as it became Africa's biggest epidemic. During the anti-apartheid struggle, this was perhaps a necessary displacement. As the comedian and HIV educator Pieter-Dirk Uys put it:

> With apartheid on our plate, there could be no other issues on the menu that demanded attention. Locals saw the HIV epidemic as something far away, in a hemisphere across the globe ... No one knew anyone suffering from AIDS. It was always somewhere else. Always somewhere far away.
>
> (Uys, 2002: 42)

Apartheid produced its own painful silencings, powerfully evoked in the literature of the time, for instance, in Bloke Modisane's poem 'lonely', an extract from which begins this chapter.[9] To struggle against another silence may have seemed impossible. At the end of the millennium, though, health minister Nkosozana Zuma castigated the 'silent epidemic' that let Gugu Dlamini die (Department of Health, 1998). Nelson Mandela (2000), speaking at the 2000 Durban AIDS Conference, called for people to 'break the silence, banish stigma and discrimination, and ensure total inclusiveness within the struggle against AIDS'. By the time of our research, people were starting to talk about HIV and demand HIV services. Representationally, there was a whole world of HIV talk out there, in TV edutainment such as *Soul City,* talk shows like *Felicia,* initiatives by national and local government and NGOs, activist campaigns posing disclosure as resistance, and oceans of coverage in newspapers and magazines. Three of our research participants had contributed to such public talk through media interviews. Yet sometimes, all this talk seemed to be doing nothing. Many people were still living with the condition in fearful silence, or with an openness that stigmatised and excluded them. None of our interviewees – even those who had appeared on television – found disclosure easy. Most had talked about their HIV status much less, and to fewer people, than they wanted.

As Uys describes it, fear and shame continued to maintain silences around HIV in the 'new' South Africa:

> President Nelson Mandela said the words, 'Never, never and never again shall it be that this beautiful land will again experience the oppression of one by another'. I knew he was right. As long as we are still alive and sane enough to remember how terrible the fear was, it can never happen again! I was wrong. It has happened again! Today the fear is worse than in those terrible days. Whereas apartheid became the banner to rally the people, AIDS is the shame to scatter the people.
>
> (Uys, 2002: 47–8)

Judge Edwin Cameron, a major figure in the anti-apartheid struggle, kept his HIV diagnosis a secret for 15 years. In *Witness to AIDS* (2005a), he writes of the 'epidemic of silence' in South Africa and of people 'looking for a voice' – one that he as a white gay man only partly provided for them (see also Cameron, 2005b: 25). Cathy Campbell describes, in the quotation that begins this chapter, the continuing externalising of HIV at every level onto other people, other localities, other agencies and institutions.

Hélène Joffe's research shows how, in the UK, South Africa and Zambia, young people in cities, women and men, black and white, 'other' their epidemics (Joffe, 1997; Joffe and Bettega, 2003). They draw on existing and new versions of xenophobia (Harris, 2002) to locate HIV on continents and among 'outsider' groups with whom they do not identify. Joffe suggests that this 'othering' preserves people's representations of their individual and social identities. Interviewees in our research retrospectively described very similar representations of HIV as a problem from and for elsewhere. Mhiki, for instance, thought herself exempt because she had not been promiscuous and had not had a partner from outside South Africa: 'I had no boyfriend from overseas and the truck drivers'. HIV's fatality and sexually transgressive associations also, as we saw in Chapter 1, accorded ill with the new South Africa's hopes for the future and resonated with the racism of apartheid and colonialism. It appeared, practically and ideologically, as an undermining of the new democracy within which people were finally speaking up after the apartheid 'years of silence', through for instance the Truth and Reconciliation Commission (Gobodo-Madikizela, 2003). How could that new democracy also speak about these new unspeakable things?

HIV's 'othering' seems strongly related to stigma, an often-assumed, rarely analysed companion of the pandemic. Stigma reduction is a proclaimed goal of HIV programmes at every level. Stigma itself is most generally taken to be, as Goffman (1963) described it, any 'undesired difference' that reduces social acceptance by being linked with a negative, usually morally suspect, social identity. Stigmata of 'discredit' attaches to those with obvious 'undesired differences', like, for instance, the thinness of AIDS. But stigmata can also be 'discreditable' – social as well as physical – when they are only potentially revealable, as with, for example, the HIV positive status of a 'healthy'-looking person. Clearly there are many forms of HIV discredit and discreditability, related to illness and death, infectiveness and contagion, sexual 'promiscuity' and 'perversion', social exclusion and religious transgression. But once these are spelled out, stigma itself can be taken apart; stigma starts to become an effect, rather than an agent. Discredit and discreditability can be undone through treatment, condom provision and education, which make the HIV positive person relatively healthy and healthy-looking, allowing them to live and work, have relationships and children, and not transmit HIV, as well as rendering them moral citizens, not sexually abnormal or punished by God.[10] At the same time, some aspects of discredit and discreditability require larger shifts in religious and social beliefs, towards less punitive ideas about faith, and non-prescriptive constructions of sexualities, particularly women's sexualities (Ratele and Shefer, 2002). As many South African commentators now argue, such changes do not imply a desertion of African cultural forms but rather a development of them.[11]

Our interviewees' stories managed to narrate stigma in ways that undid it, without glossing over it. They turned interviewees away from silence and death, towards claiming speech and life as HIV positive citizens.

Acceptance and belief

Conventionally, intimate disclosure stories follow a path that starts from ignorance or uncertainty about the problematic identity. In the case of HIV, this might involve not having heard of the virus, or thinking that it exists only elsewhere or cannot affect you. Narratives then proceed through suspicion, fear and doubt – engendered by, for instance, one's own or others' illnesses, your own 'unsafe' behaviour, or the general HIV situation in the neighbourhood or nation – to knowledge, acceptance and action.[12] A positive HIV antibody test might seem a lot clearer signifier of knowledge than those that mark, for instance, the processes of discovering gay or lesbian identity; but it can still be disregarded or disbelieved. HIV knowledge may also come less formally, through your own, your partner's or your child's physical state. In any case, knowledge and acceptance are rarely the same thing. Often, the two are separated by elements of disbelief, sadness, anger, rejection or 'denial'. Sociologists of health and illness suggest that such powerful biographical disruption (Bury, 1982) is followed by a variably complex path towards integration and reconstruction, often involving some time when the 'new' aspect of identity is foregrounded before it later becomes a more 'normalised' part of people's lives (Carricaburu and Pierret, 1995). Plummer argues that such foregrounding can lead to interpretive and political communities as the newly owned identity is 'told out' in wider and wider contexts. At times, these steps are told – and followed – in different orders, with omissions or diversions (Bury, 2001; Ciambrone, 2001), and their paths may not always be individualised or structured temporally. Given South Africa's continuing HIV treatment deficit, for example, 'normalised' HIV identities are unlikely to develop. Moreover, the country's high prevalence, and its history of 'othering' and silencing HIV, make 'speaking out' to build interpretive communities, rather than individual acceptance, particularly salient.

The story of coming to ownership though acceptance and belief was common, fully told and strongly emphasised in research participants' accounts. Many narratives reached a kind of halfway ending with phrases such as 'and then I believed' or 'at last I accepted it'. The Xhosa word translated as 'acceptance' has connotations of welcoming, as when you 'accept' someone into your house. In this research it seemed to carry this positive and powerful connotation into its use in South African English. Thus 'acceptance' was an assumption of HIV ownership that took apart the stigma of HIV, unpicking its fatality and transgressiveness, taking it into one's life. 'Belief', in Xhosa as in English a word with religious connotations, similarly undid HIV's otherness, confirming the speakers as members of a 'faith community' that understood about HIV.

In interview segments dealing with acceptance and belief, HIV was generally named and owned, in phrases such as, 'he said that I have HIV' or 'I accepted that I am HIV positive'. This inscription of ownership was repeated on the written demographics forms where a number of research participants, instead of simply ticking 'HIV positive' as their status, wrote, in English or Xhosa, 'I have it' or 'I am HIV positive'. People were, though, clear about noting aspects of non-acceptance and disbelief, especially around the shocking moment of diagnosis,[13] and explicitly naming your relation to the virus was not essential to acceptance. Interviewees commonly talked indirectly about HIV as 'this thing', both with the colloquial imprecision 'thing' has in Xhosa and English, and as a way of conferring an added distance, as in 'the big thing' or 'this thing that is spoken about'.[14] Metaphorical representations of illness are common (Sontag, 2001; Staiano, 1992), and metaphor may have particular significance in some African languages, particularly for women. HIV/AIDS has also generated new realms of creative indirection.[15] Such distancing does not equate with paralysis of action. However, speaking directly of HIV was presented by many interviewees as a mark of acting on and against the epidemic.

Some interviewees had an HIV history that mirrored that of the epidemic in the country, involving diagnosed or suspected positive status in the early or mid-1990s, denial and concealment. In this period, tragedy and fatality often overwhelmed any possibility of acceptance, as Andiswa described:

> **Andiswa**: We used to talk about it with friends, 'if I could learn that I have HIV what would I do?' The other one would say, 'Oh I would kill myself', maybe the other one would say, 'Oh I would get myself hit by a train because I am going to die anyway, instead of enduring those pains and being confined to bed', you see. Rather than people seeing me with AIDS, it's better if you find out that you have HIV to kill yourself the same day with whatever. So, that is what I thought before I learnt that I have HIV.

Such powerfully negative collective representations combined with frightening experiences of others' illnesses. Zukiswa told of not returning for test results, because she saw a dying friend:

> **Zukiswa**: So just before I went to get my results, just when I started hearing about this AIDS thing, I saw a friend of mine and she was disappearing before my eyes, just while I was waiting for the results. She made me realise that I was not ready to know, that I should rather forget about the results.

Test results, however, did not determine acceptance. Michael, as we saw in Chapter 1, ignored them. He continued his story through two further periods of illness, until his retest in 2000, in a situation of much higher public HIV awareness:

> **Michael**: The results came back positive OK, the guy told me 'No what you, say what you say to me, what you told me {that Michael tested

HIV positive before}, it's really like that'. OK I told him, 'No I want to see it physically don't tell me like that you know /mhm/ show me the paper, the papers you know, let me see it, you should see that the man is HIV positive', OK it was fine. 'How do you feel now?' now I started to become shock now, I looked up the sky like that, I looked up the sky, the guy asked me 'How do you feel?'. 'No, I mean I'm just OK' you know, but there's that question in my mind.

Michael, despite all his preparation, is shocked. Demonstrating this, he describes himself speaking in the third person – 'the man is HIV positive' – and demanding to see the paper where the result was written. When this indelible evidence of his status hit him – 'I started to become shock now, I look up at the sky' – he repeats his look of appeal. He then describes coming to acceptance through dialogues with his medical practitioner, his girlfriend and himself. The doctor tells him he can live long and well, and must be himself. His girlfriend says their relationship should continue as it was; she turns out to be positive alongside him. He narrates himself as coming to own the virus through this joint acceptance as well as his own belief, 'we two, we, we now, Michael and his girlfriend are HIV positive'.

Another route to HIV acceptance began with the interviewee's, a child's or partner's illness or death. During the late 1990s, Sylvia had a series of worsening health problems. In hospital, she was asked to take an HIV test:

Sylvia: I agreed with pleasure because I had not thought about that thing, I had no problem with it. The blood was then drawn {tested}; when the results came back, they didn't tell me directly. Instead, the doctor who had been draining me {kidney drainage} was the one who came and had a chat with me . . . He then asked me a question: 'How would you feel if you were to hear that you perhaps have a problem like HIV?'. I looked him in the face. I then said to him, 'There is nothing I would do in that situation.' He didn't tell me anything, he simply went. On the following day, a lady who is a social worker at {hospital name} and who stays around {township name} came to me. She came straight to my bed. I smiled whilst she was on her way to me as I thought she had been sent from my house for something. We had a chat . . . She then said, 'There is a problem that I want to tell you but I want you to take it easy.' I then asked what was that. My mind was convinced that I had a problem now that I was weak. After she had told me about that thing, I asked her, 'Oh no! How could this happen and where do you get this {information} from?'. She said from the doctors who were inspecting me. She also said, 'Didn't the doctor who conducted a blood test with you not tell you of what happened?'. I said, 'He came the previous day and he was trying to tell me because he asked me the same question, as to how would I feel if I were HIV positive. I answered him by saying there was nothing I would do about that, now that it was in me.' She then said, 'Yes sister it's like that.' She told me to hold tight {be strong or courageous} and, that's what I really did.

This was chronologically a much sharper path towards HIV acceptance than Michael's. Sylvia did not know anyone with HIV and only retrospectively considered her weakness a sign. She talked indirectly about the virus throughout her interview.[16] She quotes the doctor's own specific, but hedged, specification, '*perhaps* . . . a problem *like* HIV' (my emphasis) – then she looks him 'in the face' and says she will accept it. But she does not mention acceptance, but rather uses a negative formulation of acceptance's obverse, saying twice, 'there was nothing I would do'. Here, as when a number of interviewees reported doctors and nurses telling them not to 'do anything' after diagnosis, 'do' means 'do something to oneself', to kill oneself. For many South Africans, as we heard from Andiswa, this was the imagined or planned reaction to getting an HIV positive diagnosis.[17] Our interviewees most often represented it through accounts of themselves or others thinking of or actually throwing themselves under trains or swallowing household cleaners. Sylvia, however, reports herself saying she will continue to live with this potentially fatal illness – an implicit acceptance of it into her life. She also describes herself actively taking on the nurse's imperative to 'hold tight', 'that's what I really did'.

Other research participants came to HIV testing, acceptance and belief because they were worried about their health or had had unsafe sex, because VCT and some treatments were available, because they wanted to know their status – or some combination of these. Many women interviewees were diagnosed during pregnancy, taking the test because they knew MTCT treatment was likely to ensure a negative baby. Zoleka, pregnant just before the onset of the province-wide MTCT programme, tested simply because she wanted to know. The day before our interview, her baby had tested negative:

> **Zoleka**: When I was pregnant last year, that is year 2000, I went to book at the clinic. They said three types of blood tests were conducted. But, the third one was not compulsory. I told myself that I wanted to do the third test too, so as to see if I do have this thing . . . I was told I'm HIV positive. Now, after they had tested me, they told me they were going to draw another blood from my finger to check again. They tested again and told me 'yes, it's like that'. I didn't get shocked that much, just a little bit. I told myself, I wasn't going to tell anybody. I would keep it to myself, right inside. Not even my husband, and I did just that for three months.

Zoleka's husband, as we saw in the preceding chapter, accused her of 'bringing it'. She was planning on telling her sister, but had so far come to accept her status primarily through her support group:

> **Zoleka**: They {clinic nurses} introduced us to {facilitator name}. Then we kept attending the support group and also coming to take the milk powder. We would be here at 11am and chat. To those who were {newly} arriving we would ask them and show them that, 'we were once like this. We have become strong. We have accepted this thing'. That was how we {friends} met.

Zoleka's usual indirectness is broken only at the owning moment of diagnosis, when she says she was told 'I'm *HIV positive*' (my emphasis). Afterwards, it is confirmed that 'it's like that', and that 'we have accepted this thing'. She was shocked, but 'just a little bit'. She tells of her acceptance and strength through her own internal dialogues and, later, through her exchanges in the support group, in particular with the newly arriving women to whom, alongside others in the support group, she performs – and reperforms for us – acceptance and strength: 'We have become strong. We have accepted this thing.'

Perhaps post-test counselling demanded 'acceptance' too rapidly. However, many interviewees' narrated achievement of at least provisional acceptance after the test, represented powerfully both the other demands in their lives, and the demands of HIV itself, which if not accepted, would kill you. As Ntomboxolo put it, 'one must accept HIV immediately'. Sometimes, acceptance had precursors – instances of illness, testing, or thinking about testing that preconstructed an imagined HIV 'community' to which participants already to an extent belonged. Acceptance too, was, not a perfect achievement in the stories; aspects of HIV that could never be 'accepted' were included. Many interviewees, like Michael, looking up at the sky, reported a sense of deracination or strangeness after diagnosis, as if the world had shifted shape. As Ntomboxolo says at the beginning of the chapter, you might feel 'like somebody else'. These accounts of an uncanny feeling – what Freud (1925) called *unheimlichkeit* – marked how the reality of HIV hit people in a powerful, indescribable way. Later dialogues in the stories, within interpretive communities of HIV understanding constituted by medical professionals, support groups, families, and sometimes just within the interviewees themselves, built HIV ownership more strongly, managing to familiarise even this shock.

HIV interpretive communities

Medical communities

In the examples above, dialogues with others, in medical and support group 'interpretive communities', built acceptance and belief. These 'communities' treated interviewees as HIV positive citizens who could live normal, mostly healthy lives, being productive and having relationships, though also having specific health requirements. They could be open about their status, accepted by others and could educate others to ensure a citizenry as HIV-aware as they. In these support communities, HIV's ownership was collectively nego-tiated, rather than individually assumed. Our research participants provided some highly detailed narratives of their paths within such communities towards a fuller ownership of HIV.

Medical HIV communities were especially important in accounts of the period after diagnosis. By 2001, in specialist HIV medical settings, inter-viewees could assume HIV acceptance and belief, and speak of the virus without fear or discrimination. In the immediate aftermath of testing, such communities could be critical. Bulelwa, for instance, moved away from her suicidal thoughts through doctors' and nurses' encouragement:

> **Bulelwa**: Look now we are strong because of the doctors and nurses. If they hadn't encouraged us maybe we would have done those things we were thinking of when we were first told. They encouraged us, we got stronger, we are able to live with it and accept it. If they were not around maybe I would have committed suicide because I was thinking about committing suicide.

In earlier years, some interviewees had turned medical interpretive communities into their long-term HIV 'home'. Interviewees diagnosed or entering treatment more recently, told of medical professionals and coun-sellors directing them towards family members or support groups that could constitute longer-term HIV communities:

> **Benjamin**: When I went there {HIV clinic} I met Sister {name} and Doctor {name} . . . Then I introduce myself to them and then it's where I found the home for my treatment you see /mhm/ I talk to them openly. That was the first time /mhm/ to be in a, HIV positive clinic. Then from there I was introduced to a support group /mhm/ where we used to go and share our problems, like at home.

In these stories, medical professionals help patients work against stigmatisation and the sadness of living with fatal illness, addressing them as moral and social subjects. Sipho described nurses as showing an ideal form of humanity:

> **Sipho**: The nurses . . . were showing *ubuntu* {humanity}. They would chat with you so that you wouldn't be a person who thinks too much. They advise you how to do certain things.

As we saw in the previous chapter, this encouragement could extend to providing practical help such as food and forms of work, or helping with disclosure and relationships. Such boundary transgressions endorsed inter-viewees' re-valuing of themselves as HIV positive subjects who were still social and ethical citizens.

There might be problems with such a medicalised HIV community. Medical practitioners' power over HIV treatment and other resources, including HIV discourse itself, as well as their more general cultural power, could work to control their patients' stories and understandings. However, in situations of high HIV prevalence, divisions between patients and medical experts erode. Many medical professionals are themselves HIV infected or affected, as interviewees noted. The potential sharing of concerns appeared to encourage our interviewees' claiming of HIV ownership within medical communities.

There are blurrings between what doctors, nurses, counsellors and, sometimes, group facilitators do in relation to HIV, so that interpretive communities pragmatically ebbed and flowed to take in some or all of these figures at different times in the interviews. Like bell hooks (hooks and West, 1991), interviewees took their 'community' where they could find it. Counselling was, as we have heard, most often associated with diagnosis, and involved either induction into other forms of HIV 'community', or in some circumstances, advice about keeping HIV to oneself and coming to terms with it through dialogue with yourself, in a community of one. For some, counselling offered talk about HIV too early or briefly, at a time when only the diagnosis's shock could be felt, or when HIV 'belief' was partial. Mhiki for instance 'got sick with' the counselling because she thought she had no risk factors; later, by the time of the interview, she felt it could be useful. For others, counselling was an important 'encouragement' and first step towards HIV community. Some even described test counsellors as like 'mothers' in the intimate comfort they offered at this point in their HIV trajectory. The small number of interviewees who returned to their counsellors with later HIV-related problems were able to constitute this service as a constant, affirmative, though infrequently used listening 'community'. Such provision is likely to continue to be of significance around difficult events such as long-term ARV use (Stenson *et al.*, 2005) and the deaths of children, even as the HIV 'interpretive community' within neighbourhoods expands.

Support group 'families'

Support groups were a general element in stories of HIV community. Outside the hierarchies and institutional constraints of professional–client relations, yet providing, like them, HIV knowledge and understanding, they shared useful information about HIV positive living, and strengthened acceptance where it wavered. Ntomboxolo described how doubts were resolved within groups, for instance, around HIV's origins:

> **Ntomboxolo**: Like a discussion about HIV just crops up when we talk, like when we are listening to the news on the radio and they talk about HIV, maybe someone has died of HIV, like there is this kid

who said, 'Oh no girl, this HIV, where on earth did it come from?' and a discussion will start from there. And then we would realise that it's actually a disease that is spread by humans.

Groups were represented as constructing a shared sociality within which you are a person like others. You make friends, and share information and feelings. Ntomboxolo stressed, in her story of a typical session that begins this chapter, the groups' openness, dialogues, enjoyment and commonality: 'we will sit and chat and have fun'. The support group's interpretive community was often compared to family:

> **Phumla**: The first thing I noticed there, we are all happy for each other. We treat each other as we are children born of the same parents. For instance if I say I have nothing at home, one would pop out maybe R5 and say 'here take it', and they do the same if someone will speak out and say 'I do not have something to eat at home'. And we will never gossip about one another outside, no one talks about another person. We live like we are children of the same family. That is what I liked.

Where HIV positive mothers in high-prevalence epidemics report having difficulties, these seem likely to be related to lack of peer support, particularly in regard to formula feeding (Nuwagaba-Biribonwoha *et al.*, 2006).

Interviewees from the MTCT programmes almost all loved their groups and recounted many ingenious stories they had invented to explain why they were formula feeding – as Bulelwa said 'we tell lots of stories'. Such narrative resourcefulness was a good example of the groups' value in negotiating HIV within daily lives. The groups' sociality could also be carried outside, to make you more at home in the wider HIV-affected world – and even to make you healthier, more of a physical as well as social presence:

> **Zukiswa**: Even when I was pregnant I was light in weight, I was not doing alright because I would think about this {HIV} all the time even when I am just sitting at home, but that all changed when I went to the group. Even now when I walk on the streets I do not feel small {ashamed} because it might happen that s/he {others} has it but they do not know.

Participants also represented groups as places where they planned wider disclosures, further steps on the path towards openness and health. Linda, for instance, who we heard in the previous chapter describing her insistent HIV testimony to her husband, prefaced that account with a statement about her own knowledge and acceptance of HIV. She then moved to a tale of acceptance and openness in a support group that also directed her towards a wider interpretive community. The story was ordered by its personal and social significance, not chronologically: Linda put her own knowledge and acceptance first, followed by that of her husband. But in fact, the support groups were her first interpretive community, the place where she first felt 'free' and 'happy' as an HIV positive person. Moreover, at both the causal centre of the story and its chronological beginning, is the material resource that generated the group and made her husband able to listen, the MTCT programme. While treatment resources do not automatically connect to disclosure (Skogmar *et al.*, 2006), people's perceptions of such resources – in particular, those associated with healthy children – may do.

> **Linda**: Okay! In the first place I am glad I know of my HIV positive status because now I know what to do. My husband, the one I am married to, I told him. At first, he could not accept it, he gave me too many problems. I then continued talking about it every day, I used to chat about it so that it would sink into him that I am a person who is HIV positive. /mhm/ Truly, eventually he accepted it. It was before my baby was discharged yet, so that s/he could be tested as well /Okay!/ Then he asked about the baby. I said the baby will be tested at nine months. I then explained. Truly then I was told that the baby, I was very happy, because I was happy to save my baby. AZT helped me, my baby was tested negative. That made me a very happy person, I didn't think of myself as having HIV because I am still alright. There is no difference I must say. My health is still good. The other thing that made me happy is the group support that we are doing as nursing mothers. /mhm/ It really really helped us because you feel free when you are there I must say. You become very happy and forget that eish, when you get home it is then that you remember that you have HIV, but when you are there you are free. We advise each other very well, even the instructor {facilitator}, I must say she tells us what to do, so today I am not ready, I am not yet free, I don't feel like I am open, I am not open yet to stand up and say I have HIV. I will keep trying, you understand? /Mhm[18]

Linda had not yet disclosed widely – 'I am not ready' she said – but like many interviewees she saw even disclosure's planning as significant. A few interviewees treated disclosure on a 'need-to-know' basis. More presented it, like Linda, as a means to promote health, and as a self- and community-development issue. Disclosure narratives were ubiquitous and powerful in the interviews, and support groups were frequently presented as a practice ground.

Though in this study joint interviews were only one-tenth the size of support groups, they had something of a support group feel, with two or three interviewees, one or two researchers, often some babies and toddlers, and refreshments for all. Sometimes, narratives of the group interpretive community were enacted in the interviews, performing HIV ownership for the researchers and the potential broader audience, and perhaps to some degree re-establishing it for the research participants themselves. For example, Nosipho, Mandisa and Amanda collectively narrated their healthy eating procedures, originating from nurses and counsellors, but owned here through their own dialogue:

> **Amanda**: For example I did not know that if you have HIV you are not supposed to eat spicy food. I did not know that, and acid drink you are not supposed to drink it. I heard that from the clinic, we get information here/Okay/ on that side.
>
> . . .
>
> **Mandisa**: And meat. Your meat, when you cook the meat that you buy from the stands, red meat, you must cook it very well and make sure that it is well done without blood. And your fruit, you must rinse it before you eat it.
>
> **Amanda**: And your vegetables must not be overcooked.
>
> **Mandisa**: Mhm.
>
> **Amanda**: You must cook your cabbage with water.
>
> **Mandisa**: With water.
>
> **Amanda**: It must not be overcooked and lose the vitamins.
>
> **Mandisa**: Mhm.
>
> **Nosipho**: Like there is some potato, a Xhosa potato.
>
> **Mandisa**: Ingongwe.
>
> **Nosipo**: Ingongwe, do you know it?
>
> **Interviewer**: No, no.
>
> **Nosipho, Mandisa, Amanda**: African potato {in English}.
>
> **Interviewer**: Okay.
>
> **Nosipho**: We get told about it, that you must use it, mix it with garlic and ginger, use a grater and boiling water. Like do not cook them, put boiling water in a bottle and add the mixture. Every morning take half a cup every morning. Maybe if you do not have appetite you will gain appetite and your blood will be alright.

Co-constructed stories of this kind were persuasive demonstrations by the research participants of themselves as members of powerful, active HIV support communities.

Research participants interviewed individually also often 'performed' interpretive community. Ntomboxolo, for example, told the story of the induction of women into the support group community of HIV positive citizens, through an elaborate solo 'performance' of the group. This story had a primary place in Ntomboxolo's interview; it was the first thing she told us. She was also one of the few interviewees who said she could not safely tell any family members or friends her status. The support group seemed likely, then, to continue to be a particularly powerful HIV community for her, and she represented it to us – and herself – in a specially effective way:

Ntomboxolo: Oh no, there's nothing wrong with the support group, it's like the best thing, we sit and chat. For instance if there's a new beginner, we as the old members, we would not be able to talk to strangers, then counsellor {facilitator name} would give us the go ahead, so that we can ask the new person for details.

The new member would greet us and ask how do we do?

The old members would respond, and then tell {facilitator name} that we cannot talk freely in front of the new faces, so {facilitator name} would say, 'Go on ask her for details', she does not talk, only we do the talking.

We would ask, 'Sister what are you doing here?'

She would probably say, she came to fetch the milk formula for the baby.

We would say 'This is not the place to fetch milk formula, why do you have to get milk formula?'

She would say, 'I do not breast-feed.'

We would ask, 'Why are you not giving breast milk to your baby?'

She would maybe say, 'I'm ill'.

We would ask, 'Which illness?'

Then she would not say.

And then we would say, 'Then we ask you to please leave the room if you do not want to tell us why you are not breast-feeding your child.'

Sometimes, other women ask the new beginners, 'At the time when they drew {tested} your blood, what were you told is in your blood?'

Then the other beginner would tell us, 'They told that I am HIV positive so that's why I can't give breast milk to my baby', then we would let her stay.

And then we would move on to the next one, let's say we have about three of them.

Then we would ask the third one, 'And you Sisi, what are you doing here?'.

May be she would just open up easily and say, 'I am HIV positive'.

So then we would ask, 'How did it feel when you were told for the first time in the clinic after they took your blood sample and told you that you are positive?'.

Some women usually say, 'I felt alright.'

'Who did you tell?'.

One would probably say, 'My husband,' and maybe the other one say, 'My parents.'

Do you get the picture?[19]

Both in joint and individual interviews, then, the research itself seemed to offer an opportunity to rehearse and perhaps strengthen people's representational strategies for owning HIV, by revisiting support groups' 'interpretive community'.

The group's only requirement, as Ntomboxolo described, is to start from the open acknowledgement that 'we are all HIV positive'; and from confidentiality. But support groups were not always inclusive. As we heard in Chapter 3, some facilitators were thought more including than others. Some interviewees, like Benjamin, remained silent when they first attended, testing the group out, not wanting to say much about themselves, just listening. Silent participation was still an important form of participation but facilitators would on occasion talk to such group members separately, eliding group support with individual counselling, as one of the research gatekeepers described:

> **Nomakuthweni**: OK, my role in the group is sometimes to share their problem. So I make someone, she does not want to say, because the room is full, she meets me outside/I see/ so that person comes out to tell me a problem. So I think it's my role.

Sometimes the groups' heterogeneity was problematic. Nosizwe, now a strong part of her support group, thought initially that women in the group were, by virtue of their openness and cheerfulness, different from her – immoral:

> **Nosizwe**: Here, when I got here it was worse. I got here to people that were not worried, they were happy, they even seemed silly. When I first got here it was not nice for me. I came back again and then I tried to adjust and I then realised that no they are not being silly, it is because they have accepted the support group. I found advice here and if something is troubling you for example you talk about your boyfriend and the way he doesn't care about you. Here you'd get here and find people with the same problem and then you would be able to perservere.

Men's lesser access to groups made some feel 'left out' of the ownership of HIV information. Sipho ended his story of searching for a support group with a request to talk to a social worker in order to find one. However, HIV 'ownership' within groups is always imperfect and changing. Groups with full knowledge of ARVs were rare at the time of the research. Other uncertainties arose later as group concerns, for instance, around ARVs' long-term side-effects, and secondary ARV regimes. The ownership offered by groups could, conversely, be overwhelming; Zola said he felt like a newcomer in the HIV world, not yet ready to find out about viral load and ARVs. Yet most interviewees said they wanted to know everything they could, and saw the groups as a route to such knowledge. David, the only interviewee who explicitly mentioned people with serious illnesses attending support groups, wanted to include these HIV community members too within his understanding:

> **David**: {In the groups}, yes, when I see a person who is ill who is HIV
> positive. It makes me aware that even myself I will be I will be sick,
> I mean I don't know but I am a very strong person. I'm aware of
> everything, I know I will be sick.

Our interviewees' stories of the groups thus balanced the groups' divisions
and imperfections of knowledge and inclusiveness, against the collective
HIV understandings they developed within them.

It is important to remember that stories are strongly determined by material
circumstances. Linda's story of MTCT treatment, and those of many other
women, indicate the importance of perceived effective treatment for intimate
disclosure narratives. The availability of travel money, food and income-
generation projects, as well as treatment resources, also helped construct
support groups as interpretive communities. Yet support groups also work
independently of material provision. They have been key resources for
attaining HIV ownership in situations where few medical resources are
available – in the early days of the US, UK and Ugandan epidemics, for
instance. For many of our research participants, medical treatment was scant,
but collective talk was represented as a resource in itself, something that kept
people healthy – a pragmatic necessity for positive HIV life.

In South Africa, as in many other HIV contexts, the policy assumption is
that people will 'move on' from support groups into wider support communities. By 2001, two years after her diagnosis, Yoliswa found support
groups' concerns irrelevant. Benjamin, diagnosed in the early 1990s, had
moved from support groups into activism. Michael, who had attended
support groups a year before, was now facilitating groups himself. By
2003–4, most of the research participants who had been in support groups in
MTCT prevention programmes were either living in their neighbourhoods
with no contact with HIV services, were providing those services themselves,
or were participating in income-generation projects orientated towards
HIV positive people. In the developed world, HIV support group 'micro'-
communities have developed as the epidemic progresses, with groups for
the newly diagnosed, those starting ARVs, long-term survivors, and demographic sectors such as gay men, drug users, women and people of African
origin. While support groups in South Africa may also become more
specialised in the kinds of viral 'ownership' they offer, here, the general
population constitutes the largest HIV 'community'. Most of that community
is living with the condition in similarly resource-constrained conditions.

Support groups seem likely, nevertheless, to remain an important form of
HIV community within South African civil society. Though they may seem
like a new and 'western' resource, they resemble other forms of South
African community organisation such as residents' and savings associations
and church groups, especially women's church groups. Like church groups,
they focus on building collective understanding, as well as providing the
shared intimacy and mutual responsibility that characterise the other groups.

For people like Ntomboxolo, they were a continuing necessity. But some interviewees with strong family support were also long-term support group members. Mary, whose family knew her HIV status, was still with her group in 2004 and was something of a role model for it, living healthily, on ARVs, active in HIV campaigns, and doing much of the group's practical work such as keeping records and distributing donated food and clothes.

Most interviewees planned to extend the ownership of HIV they had found in support groups. Some told of intragroup friendship networks that now took in other activities – for instance, going to church. While they were practising disclosure in the groups in order to move outward into wider HIV communities of family and friends, they could also use the groups to move 'back' to medical support:

> **Zukiswa**: You would then get pills and medicines, like for those that are, who have severe effects from it {HIV}. A person from the group, you can see them and they will also notice if they are getting sick and speak to counsellor {facilitator name} and then go see the doctor.

Support group narratives of HIV understanding were thus, as policy-makers and educators hoped they would, enabling people with HIV to extend their interpretive communities more widely, but also to establish a conduit to appropriate medical treatment for the future.[20]

Family and neighbourhood communities

Most research participants described efforts to construct familial 'communities' of HIV understanding. Interviewees told stories of going home from support groups or clinics and using the language of these HIV interpretive communities to tell partners and relatives what they had found out. Busisiwe, for example, described taking her understanding of safe sex from the groups to her boyfriend and other friends:

> **Busisiwe**: What I say is that 'you see I don't beg you'. I say, 'You my dearest friend, there are only the two of us here, we must use a condom because a condom would help us because I won't be around when you are sleeping with another girl. So, you wouldn't even know what disease that girl has besides HIV, you would sleep with her and then come to sleep with me which would add on the disease I already have, what I have would multiply, yet if you are using a condom, it's important.' He then said that I must come with the whole plastic {bag} full of condoms, then I was thrilled . . . so I persuade {friends} to use condoms otherwise to do nothing. One day I was opening my brother's bag, and when I look through his stuff, 'Wow! Lots of condoms!'.

This storied construction of an unambiguously condom-positive HIV 'community' of partner, friends and siblings was unusually explicit and straightforward. Such tales were usually, as we saw in the previous chapter, interwoven with detailed considerations of why people reacted or might react well or badly, on the basis of, for instance, religious beliefs, character factors such as drinking and gossiping, family histories of illness or conflict, and generationally different approaches to sexuality, particularly women's sexuality. Even for Busisiwe, HIV community was sometimes hard to negotiate within her family. Early on in her interview, she describes her mother's ambivalent acceptance and the words of her HIV negative sister helping to establish an HIV familial 'community':

> **Busisiwe**: My mum said when she was talking to me, 'I will take you in, both you and this HIV live in this house.' My sister . . . said, 'Don't take in this child if you don't accept that she has HIV, don't push her away, accept her, take her, look after her as your child that you gave birth to. There are many other diseases like rheumatism, diabetes and the like, things that are similar to this incurable thing. So, please, do not discriminate against her, so take her in, mould her, make her your child, do not discriminate against her.'

But her mother's insults continue. Busisiwe tells of returning to the support group community which she uses to model her HIV citizenship, and then going back to her family, trying again to include them in her HIV community:

> **Busisiwe**: So when these insults come, I just want to go to the group for a chat . . . This {support group} is how I am these days when I'm with my family, 'people we must accept this because there is no one who will be uninfected by this thing forever'. In that way I know that I want them to know that it does not pick certain people over others.

Busisiwe's story represents her as strongly committed to building commonality, as an HIV positive person, with her mother, who positions her infected daughter as 'other'. Busisiwe describes sympathetically her mother's financial difficulties, her aloneness, her health problems. She believes her mother *must* accept her, 'because she knew me when I was young'. She finishes the interview with regret that her mother is still not part of her HIV 'community', one that must include 'respectable' mothers as well as 'disreputable' daughters:

> **Busisiwe**: {At the clinic} I felt bad because my mum wasn't there to see that 'all my peers are here', and actually realise that this thing does not infect only certain people.

An important set of stories dealing with the limits of HIV community addressed new mothers' explanations of formula feeding. The stories were for many interviewees important modes of negotiating their newly realised HIV status within the 'communities' of their families and neighbourhoods. While acknowledging the virus, the stories weighed disclosure's benefits, few in this case, against its potentially stigmatising effects on women and babies. The virus was 'owned' – declared, accepted and understood – in one HIV community, but also 'owned' by its concealment within another, non-HIV aware community. The stories located reasons for formula feeding in maternal medical causes, the mother's personal decision or other external circumstances – never with the baby. Ntomboxolo claimed her milk would not come out, and as this had been the case with her first child, people believed her. Zukiswa told people she had not breast-fed her first child and could not with this one owing to a 'dirty substance' that came from her breast. Though she had in fact breast-fed the first child, no one in her new and highly mobile neighbourhood knew or remembered. The trope of dirty or inadequate milk or body was deployed in many stories. Lindi said she had a breast infection; Nosizwe said some other medicines she took would harm the milk; Andiswa claimed a 'problem' with her breasts; Linda said her breasts had poison in them; Nomthandazo told people that her breasts were dry but because her husband was unemployed she was able to get free formula. Other women simply invoked their own or others' wishes. Phumla said she did not want to breast-feed; Amanda, the youngest interviewee, was told by her father to formula-feed so she could stay in school. Two women had problems with their stories. Nosipho's mother made her breast-feed until she induced her mother to visit the clinic nurse, who gave a non-disclosing explanation. Nomazwe's story of sore breasts and 'off' milk, which her baby would not take, did not convince her mother-in-law. She had to insist on the correctness of this approach against the older woman's conviction, not uncommon in such situations, that doctors don't know much about babies.

In a situation where MTCT and its early successes were widely known, where little treatment was available for HIV positive children, who often died as infants, and where HIV itself was still largely a silent matter, these stories of maternal problems and external contingencies were nuanced social negotiations. Perhaps the pathologisation of the 'poisoned', 'dry', 'dirty' and 'infected' mothers in many stories expressed some of the mothers' own concerns, persisting alongside their 'acceptance'. Perhaps it simply drew adeptly on the common cultural pattern of blaming mothers for infant problems, in order to avoid pathologising the babies, a concern found elsewhere in South Africa (Clark, 2006); the women's expressed satisfaction with their stories seemed to support this. Perhaps the issue was already partly defused by a growing implicit acceptance of the possibility of HIV among formula-feeding mothers – a form of non-disclosing acceptance to which I shall return.

Interviewees' stories of bringing friends and neighbours into their HIV communities were even more problematic. As we saw in the previous chapter, these social networks operated as HIV communities for relatively few interviewees, though proportionally more of the male interviewees mentioned them. Most frequently, interviewees told stories of assessing their friends' reactions to HIV topics prior to disclosure and realising disclosure was ill-advised:

> **Mhiki**: I don't have friends. I had a friend before. My child was sick and every time she was in the {name} hospital. My friend said to me, I didn't tell my friend I'm HIV positive, 'why your child is always sick, the best way you must just dump her in the hospital'.

Narratives of broader communities of HIV were predominantly negative, including many small stories of discrimination. The stories almost always concluded that outside your family, only the HIV-aware – for instance, those met through support groups – can be your friends. Zola went beyond this negative assessment to produce a narrative of general hostility, covering a racialised majority of the nation, and specifically identifying the HIV positive man's exclusion from productive citizenship:

> **Zola**: My people is different from other people like Coloureds or other people you see because my people if you go down, they press you down you see. They don't try to help you . . . maybe I go home and tell my people 'hey', that 'people fire me'. My people do not feel what I'm feeling. They say, 'yah you think you are clever, you don't even support us. You just say you go to work'. That's why my people is different from other people.

Many interviewees like Busisiwe told stories of talking *about* HIV with friends in ways that suggested an incipient HIV community of people ready to hear. Yet people not yet openly, knowingly or directly affected by HIV were glad of disclosure, as Pam said: 'So I accepted it, I told my friends they accept me and they like me because I didn't hide it.' Benjamin, Michael, Siphiwe and David also told stories of HIV interpretive community among friends – relatedly, perhaps, no men told stories of the sexualised shame attached to HIV positivity that appeared in many women's accounts. For these men, stories of talking about HIV with trusted friends were stories of liberation and support. David had indeed been brought into an interpretive community around HIV through his friendship with Michael, who talked openly about his status without making it define his friendships:

> **David**: I was one of those people {not wanting} to know that I'm HIV positive and er I will sit at home then maybe when I get sick that's when I went {to the clinic}. But somewhere along the way I changed my mind and the guy who really helped me with that is this guy

Michael. I mean the guy really helped me. I mean I've known him, that he was HIV positive, but we never talked about it. Then one day I decided to come here {to} this clinic and to be tested.

At this point and still today, individuals such as Michael who are open within their communities – evangelists of HIV understanding – are powerful embodiments of HIV citizenship. Michael was an exemplary figure across ages and genders, appearing in the stories of several other interviewees who had both heard and seen him in the neighbourhood, healthy and active, talking about accepting and living with HIV:

> **Busisiwe**: You see, you wouldn't believe that my brother {Michael} is HIV positive, people get shocked because he has really accepted this. So you must accept this, you must be open. I want what he also wants.

Virtual HIV communities

Those whose everyday HIV communities were limited often emphasised ways of building HIV ownership through imaginary or virtual routes. Interviewees who used the internet, the most-cited developed-world virtual community, found some HIV information through it but did not have enough access to allow them to become part of online communities, although some South Africans do participate in HIV chat rooms and message boards. Radio and television soap operas, talk shows, news reports, and newspaper and magazine features, were, however, worked into most interviewees' lives as HIV citizens. By talking about HIV, these media, like support groups, destigmatised it (Hutchinson and Mahlalela, 2006), providing accurate, helpful and hopeful information. They showed that 'there are many people with HIV, I am not alone', and that you can live long and healthily, and have good relationships. And they inducted people around you into parallel HIV ownership, as Linda and Phumla clarify in this joint narrative:

> **Linda**: It gave me hope, when I heard from the radio that people talk about it. Like, I used to say {to myself} if they talk about it, it would be like they are talking about me they are telling the people that I live with about my problem. I always hoped that the more they talk about it on the radio, the more and better understanding the people I live with will have on the day I find time to tell them, they will accept me.
>
> . . .
>
> **Phumla**: Me, everything, like if I find something like a newspaper whether it's the *Argus*, anything, as I used to work as a domestic worker, I would look out for anything that says something about HIV I would start with it and look at it and read it. The radio as well,

is very encouraging. There are many people that talked, that is what I enjoyed listening to. I would hear someone saying 'I have {HIV for} 20 years', maybe they would identify themselves. I then realised that there are many people with HIV, I am not alone. On TV they would show us everything, so that brought me hope that maybe all of us in the world will be like that. I have hope because I don't want to feel alone. The radio encouraged us, people would disclose their HIV positive status on the radio, some are married. It was mostly married people that went to the radio to disclose.

Busiswe drew considerable support from these media communities. She described watching HIV television items with the family, using them as models of how the issue should be addressed, and identifying with television figures rumoured to have HIV. She positioned public figures who had been open about their HIV involvement – Nkosi Johnson, Nelson Mandela – as exemplars for her own growing HIV ownership. She wanted to act against HIV by going public herself, to save others who thought it would not affect them. In her narrative, not just failure to disclose, but any constraint on HIV's interpretive community, makes you sick:

Busisiwe: So, I'm not afraid of this because it doesn't help even if I hide it and say 'No I am scared I won't talk about it in front of other people'. It will come out eventually that I've got it to the very people that I was hiding it from. It's better if you talk about something, {if not} you start feeling like, your body starts getting thin, a little. Unlike having to think and think, like when you talk about something you become happy, like if you haven't, there is no point in hiding it. I even asked my brother did he want to see me on TV and he said, 'I want you to go'. I said to him, 'I don't have a problem at all about talking about it because, even my sister would see me on TV and realise that "okay Busisiwe has passed this on {told people about this}". I don't have the problem of a person who would be (surprised) saying 'oh my father's child is having this'. There are many of us who are infected, we are saving those who don't have it, like the old people.

Other interviewees conceptualised virtual communities around information, rather than acceptance and disclosure. Like Benjamin reading his medical catalogues and Zukiswa taking notes from the radio, David pursued HIV knowledge by reading all the leaflets and articles he could:

David: I'm very curious about AIDS. I want all the information I can get. Yes . . . I'm really doing that {reading things}. So I'm very curious about the information related to it. I think it's going to help me to know more about this virus, you know. That's the only change in me.

Like support groups, virtual HIV communities could be overwhelming. Overcoming this difficulty was described as part of the process of coming to full HIV understanding:

> **Miranda**: It is still difficult for me to watch things like prayers {for people with HIV} on TV.
> **Khondiya**: I was just like my sister here I didn't want to accept it. I didn't want to watch it even on *Soul City*.

Virtual HIV communities could also be ambiguous. As we saw in the previous chapter, interviewees struggled to assess the legitimacy of media HIV information, particularly when cures and money were at stake. Attempts at building wide-ranging virtual communities of HIV knowledge could also come up against the specific nature of some HIV understandings. For instance, the US book on healthy living used in one support group had to be set against local material resources for such living. Here, Miranda and Khondiya raise this issue, at the same time as they describe the book:

> **Miranda**: (The book) says that that one {garlic} which comes from the ground is not very good because sometimes you don't wash it properly. So, we must buy the tablets and the tablets are very expensive, R100 a bottle.
> **Interviewer**: Who said it's not good if it comes from the ground, who said that?
> **Miranda**: The small book that we read.
> **Interviewer**: Okay, does your whole group use it?
> **Miranda**: Yes, because they {facilitator, clinic staff} say it's good for us.
> **Khondiya**: It explains you must eat this, it's alright, you mustn't eat this, it's wrong.
> **Interviewer**: You sound a bit doubtful.
> **Miranda**: Sometimes I trust, sometimes I don't know because where am I going to get that R100 because I'm not working.

Only one interviewee had disclosed her status at church. Religious institutions' reported reactions to HIV were, as we saw in the last chapter, diverse, but rarely accepting enough to engender open HIV community, though many interviewees wanted this. Sipho reported being excluded in a social way, because he was not a regular attender and didn't understand everything that went on: 'It would be better if there can be a person who visits you and explains to you what the church is all about so that you would get used to it,' he said. Faith did, however, operate as virtual community for many interviewees, through individual prayer and other personal religious experiences. Busisiwe's account of her reassuring ancestor dreams gave spiritual 'community' central place in her story, coming directly after her own acceptance of her diagnosis, before even family or friends knew:

> **Busisiwe**: Another thing that strengthened me is that I told myself that I do have HIV, and my family from underground {ancestors} and the big home {ancestral home} would constantly show the sign (lifts her beads into the shape of an AIDS ribbon) to me before I woke up even before I could rise to {her ancestor's name} they would confirm every time that 'my child you are HIV positive, you must just accept it, we are behind you'.

Communities of speech and action

Plummer suggests that 'communities' of speech and action can be closely linked. In the case of speaking out as an HIV positive citizen in South Africa, it appears that speech is rather literally a speech *act* (Searle, 1969; Butler, 1993), one that has clear effects, and that cannot easily be undone. For most interviewees, there were powerful interconnections between intimate disclosure, and other more obviously practical forms of HIV ownership.

In 2001, interviewees such as Yoliswa and Michael had moved from disclosing in support groups to being HIV activists in their neighbourhoods and the province, campaigning for treatment and other services. Benjamin had become an informal local educator and advocate, talking to young people and urging HIV positive friends to give up their secrecy and live positively. Other interviewees, such as Busisiwe and Vuyani, had moved from dialogues with themselves and their families, to speaking *about* HIV to friends and neighbours. Many wanted to speak more directly about HIV; some planned to do this while providing practical, hopefully paid help in the HIV field. Phumla narrated such associations of intimate and public HIV ownership in her future plans for her HIV positive citizenship:

> **Phumla**: What I know is, like I wish we could spread out and not stay in one place, like if maybe as we have HIV we could go out and help, even if we are given two days a month, to go out and help the {ill} people who cannot move. As we are able to stand up, we should encourage them we should even if two days per month and then they should support us with at least R100 per month. We should not remain in one place. We should try to reach out and help those people that can't do anything, save them and show them that we have HIV as well so they should have hope . . . Whether it's the sick or for instance there are {HIV positive} mothers, they can go to the pregnant women, ask for a room in the clinic you understand, then we mothers can privately speak with pregnant women and give them advice. We can encourage them and show them how to do things. So that we don't relax in one place, let me put it that way.

By 2003–4, many interviewees had indeed moved out of HIV-oriented support groups into income generation groups: home care work or education and advocacy – sometimes paid, albeit at a low level. As Phumla had suggested this sometimes involved 'mothers to mothers-to-be': women advising other women going through HIV positive pregnancies as they had. Just as speech does, these practices assumed and performed HIV ownership.

Even in 2001, for some, political action was the major form of HIV ownership, enabling personal ownership. Phumla and Linda began their interview with political stories, which framed their later-described plans:

> **Linda**: What I found helpful for me was to stand up and do something because before, coming to the group was all that I did and then sitting at home because I was scared of being seen by the people outside. So I joined an organisation that is fighting for the rights of HIV positive people. So being in their midst helped me a lot because now I can face the problems that come along with my HIV positive status. That fear of feeling alone is gone. They helped me a lot. I was also motivated to tell my family, because I stayed for a long time without informing my family and the father of my baby, I was scared.
>
> . . .
>
> **Phumla**: The reason why I joined {organization name} is because it is important for someone with HIV positive status, I realised that it is important for me to stand up and be part of the people who are fighting for people's rights, I did not want to sit down and wait for things to come to me. I realised that it is vital that I stand up and help the people that are fighting for our rights.

Communities of non-disclosing acceptance

The expansions of interpretive communities of HIV planned by many interviewees were often described as being pursued implicitly, through building communities of HIV talk, but not disclosure. These were situations of *non-disclosing acceptance* within which our interviewees suggested disclosure might happen later, when appropriate. For the interviewees recontacted in 2003 and 2004, such expansions of disclosure had indeed happened. They had told family members and, in a few cases, friends, and some were openly HIV positive in the context of voluntary or paid HIV work. They had pushed back the boundaries of HIV ownership, negotiating that ownership within wider communities. Nevertheless, non-disclosing HIV talk remains an important means of generalising HIV community in many contexts.

In 2001, communities of unspoken knowledge and acceptance were narrated by many research participants as an important partial resolution of their disclosure concerns. For Vuyani, who as we saw in Chapter 3 had found acceptance with friends at the clinic and his own family, his church constituted a non-disclosing but still significant support community. Here, HIV was discussed in general terms, and an eventual spiritual solution held out, in parallel with a medical one, sustaining Vuyani as an individual HIV positive believer:

> **Vuyani**: The other thing is that I am a believer, understand. So in church, like the Bible, we discuss about the Bible that okay, things like this happen, but it is the Devil that does these things, so we cannot give up and say 'Okay if someone has got this problem this is the end of life', you see. Well, it is God who is going to solve this problem. If we truly believe that God is alive, these things that we have, these diseases that we have are going to be cured, understand. So I mean I always have hope even when I pray. I also ask God to take this thing away from me.

More often, family and friendship networks constituted communities of non-disclosing acceptance. In Amanda's stories of her sisters and friends, for instance, undisclosed HIV is twice registered, and accepted, with simple 'oh's:

> **Amanda**: There is a woman {from the support group} that lives in my area . . . We are still also friends outside {the group}. People usually ask me at home, how did I meet up with her. I say 'no, I got to know her from fetching the milk'. They would ask why are we fetching milk, my sisters would ask 'why do you collect milk?'. I say 'no, I was told not to breast-feed because my breast milk is not good so that I can breast-feed a baby, on the other hand I don't know why she is collecting milk'. They would say 'oh'. . . . I have a friend that lives close to home, she gave birth in July. I gave birth before her and then she in July. Now when she came out of hospital, I went to see her at home with my baby. I asked her whether she breast-feeds the baby. She said no she doesn't. I then asked why, she then said no that is what she was told at the clinic, that she should not breast-feed. I then said 'oh'. I understood the reason why so I did not ask her lots of questions because I could see that she does not want to talk about it, but I know.

At a time when, in this area, up to 50 per cent of young pregnant women were testing positive, an unspoken possibility of HIV attached to formula feeding. Within their creative stories to explain such feeding, women frequently remarked their families' and friends' almost deliberate lack of interest. Mandisa's mother, for example, ignored – but accepted – her markedly precocious account:

Mandisa: I told her {mother} immediately, when I got back from {name} clinic for a booking. I got back and told her that I will not feed my baby with breast milk, I will get milk from the clinic. My mother was not interested in the details as to 'why now do you come back to tell me that you don't breast-feed, whereas you don't even have the baby yet'. She never asked too many questions, she just left it like that.

Non-disclosing talk *about* HIV could be a way of providing supportive community, as with Bulelwa, who encouraged friends to test while saying she had not, in order not to have to talk about her own status:

Bulelwa: We talk about it sometimes and I say they should get tested and I will also get tested. I want them to know . . . I think they have it.

Not mentioning HIV can be a sign of having it, as Busisiwe remarked, so talking about it might mean you are negative. Sometimes, non-disclosing support even led to a situation where interviewees lied about their status while at the same time promoting an affirmative understanding. Zukiswa, for instance, promoted testing to apparently non-HIV involved friends, by claiming she had been tested and was negative:

Zukiswa: We usually talk, but people are scared and they do not want to test their blood. I would be thinking that I know I have it. I would keep my mouth shut and tell them that it is better to get tested. They would ask whether you have been there yet. Then I would say, 'I've been there to get my blood tested and I found out that I am not positive.'

It is, of course, likely that many of Bulelwa's and Mandisa's friends were in similar positions, so that all, speakers and listeners, were in the process of generating a talking culture around HIV that developed ownership without risking stigmatisation or the difficult personal stories and questionings that may follow disclosure. As Bulelwa concluded, 'I think they have it.' This kind of talk worked to support speakers by allowing them to articulate their HIV knowledge; to educate their hearers, for many of whom it was a known or suspected problem; and to produce an implicit version of HIV community where the virus could be spoken about, albeit in the third person.

Stories of implicit HIV ownership and action through non-disclosing talk were for many participants an effective strategy for undoing HIV stigma, highly specific to their situation within this epidemic. Such non-disclosing disclosure may nevertheless appear in other contexts of stigma and epidemic. It seems to 'work' as a kind of temporary or partial resolution only within a more general cultural 'story' of expanding HIV ownership. Outside such a metanarrative, implicitness can be a mode of disowning. Like song (Guzana,

2000), gossip (Spacks, 1985) or playful language, generally, its effectiveness can be negligible, or great.[21] For someone like Busisiwe, eager to expand her story of life with HIV to wider audiences, non-disclosing acceptance was limiting. For women like Amanda, Mandisa, Bulelwa and Zukiswa, it was a significant help in their initial negotiations of HIV ownership.

Owning feelings

Coming to terms with the virus through owning it is limited by what is possible to 'own' about HIV. What could not always be 'said' within interviewees' stories were concerns about transgressions of sexual and other practice norms, loss and grief – particularly around the deaths of children – and sometimes, the 'thing', HIV, itself. For some, these 'unspeakable' concerns indicate unrepresentable emotions associated with HIV, that people's stories will inevitably gloss over or misrepresent (Craib, 2004). Alternatively, we can make double readings of people's stories that acknowledge both the resilience and the fragility that they express (Brandt, 2005). My approach, however, draws on Julia Kristeva's psychoanalytic and literary theory, as well as a number of social theorists of emotions, to argue that feelings are produced within and by structures of representation, rather than simply expressed through them.[22]

Our research participants' 'unrepresentable' concerns could be said to fall into the realm of what Kristeva calls the abject, which can be negotiated through symbolic language though not really represented by it. A territory of disgust and horror, but also of fascination and even pleasure, the abject is for Kristeva an unavoidable part of subjects' relationship to language. It is produced at the moment when the subject separates itself from its infantile physical existence and enters the social world, and thus it has a particular relation to maternity, the body and its products – blood, milk, tears, vomit – and to death, animality and 'others' who are not social subjects.[23] It is on the border between subject and object, desire and thought, death and life. Narrative language, Kristeva says, situates a person 'between desires and their prohibitions' but is also 'a thin film constantly threatened with bursting' (1984: 141) by abjection. It seems, as Young (1990: 142ff.) suggests, that the abject is drawn into play precisely at 'borders' not just of psychic but of social and historical contestation, around the condition of HIV but also around issues of 'race, gender, sexuality, age and the dis/abled body'.[24] These characteristics give abjection a double mobility. It is always to some degree apparent within language, but language continues around it. It can appear within the genre of intimate disclosure, for instance, without being fixed by that genre or breaking it up. But the abject may also move into and out of focus in relation to, for instance, HIV, as the social and historical situating of that condition shifts.

There were many occasions on which the socialised and sexualised abjection of HIV was described, and sometimes analysed, within the interviews. People told us about family members who 'accepted' their status, yet did not touch them and refused the food they cooked. Many described bodily signs that generated intense anxiety for themselves and others, such as thinness, persistent coughing and sweating. 'Poisoned' breasts or milk, could, as we saw in the case of nursing mothers, be a protective mimesis of abjection.

Women interviewees like Pam and Lindi described feeling on the borders of religious community, 'abject', between exclusion and inclusion, sometimes attending churches but not 'saved', because their status as mothers outside marriage made this impossible in the evangelical congregations that constituted their faith communities. Kristeva relates abjection to monotheism; it is the impurity and defilement against which the monotheistic religious principle, the social and political laws derived from it, and language, stand. Laws and the language that expresses them constrain lawlessness – actions that bring individual and social 'bodies' close to death – within a persecutory taxonomy that renders sexuality and women abject. To come into dialogue with laws, and the monotheistic principle from which they derive, the subject must separate from the lawless, abject body of the mother, rooted in a physicality that is indexed in the Biblical abominations of blood and milk (1984: 112), that comes close to death in childbirth, and that is tied to sexuality. This religious coding of 'feminine' abjection cannot fail to shape religious representations of women and HIV. While the control through Christianisation of African women's and men's bodies (Butchart, 1998; Hook, 2004) has been much discussed, so too have the dramatic reshapings of Christianity in Africa, particularly since the development of African churches. Women's role in these churches is very strong. These shifts, however, may not always change the abjectification by Christianity of female bodies as 'used and unclean', something that has long been recognised by African feminists (Motanyane 1987: 17). As Nosipho, an interviewee strongly connected to religious life, described it, HIV will never be a disease like others, particularly for women, because it is connected to a sexuality that is transgressive and out of synch with a measured ethical life:

Nosipho: Like the way I see people on the outside {of HIV}, I do not think that they will accept this because once people know that you have HIV they think badly about you. They think that you were sleeping around with many different people. The reason why they accepted TB is because it has nothing to do with sex, that is why they accepted it. You see HIV and AIDS have been there for a long time. They can't accept it, they think bad as in 'yho it suits her because she does not have self control, so she must have AIDS'. They interpret it negatively when you have AIDS. That is why they can't accept it.[25]

There were times in the interviews when abjection intruded directly into the frame. Pam, as we saw in Chapter 3, talked, with some difficulty, about aspects of her life such as unprotected sex and drinking that placed her outside HIV's moral 'community'. In the course of a long account, interspersed with laughs and pauses, of her difficulties with safe sex, she used the common simile of sex with a condom being like 'eating a sweet with a paper you know with a plastic, you didn't remove that'. This trope relates 'safe' sex to a sweet yet spoiled thing. The sweet is covered with a substance as unnatural to the mouth as the condom is to flesh. The conjunction invokes in the listener an almost physical irritation, a desire to get rid of this odd thing. The simile works in Pam's story, as perhaps it does in others, to say things indirectly about sexuality that are difficult to put into words. But it does not 'fix' HIV's representation fetishistically (Ahmed, 2004). It leaves it open to negotiation and change.

Words are always going to be notable failures in the face of the death of a child. Busisiwe, talking about the still-birth of her baby at four months into pregnancy, said she was as 'young' – perhaps too, as small – as the shiny new tape recorder or 'radio' we were using, gesturing to it. This material simile again represented something difficult to say, but did not derail her story, rather forcing a recognition of unrepresentable loss into the interview. Busisiwe told this story as part of her route of HIV acceptance, concluding by moving back into the representable world of HIV ownership, where her premature baby constituted proof to her of her status:

> **Busisiwe**: I discovered that I was HIV positive. I accepted it in that way. I realised that I had to accept it since I had seen both the tummy and the baby and there is nothing I can dispute.

In what looks at first like a rather different example, Yoliswa told in her interview the story of her baby's illnesses and death, a tale she had told many times in public, in support groups and to media audiences, as part of local campaigns for MTCT rollout. This repetition was a form of activism, a way of pursuing Yoliswa's expressed wish that this preventable death not happen to other children. In the interview, Yoliswa also talked at greater length about her guilt. She had known about HIV but had not used condoms because she did not take it seriously, and her baby had suffered because of this, she said several times. Such guilt might be an unexpressed element of many parents' experiences of their children's HIV-related deaths. In this case, its repetition broke up the stories, appearing almost like a material 'thing' in itself, falling out of the progressive, campaigning narrative line. Again, though, the repetition did not fix Yoliswa's feelings. They were not discharged or banalised by their representation. Nor did they work, unrepresented, to punish her, as some responses to the stigma of STIs seem to do, when for instance people use physically destructive substances such as bleach to cleanse themselves (Ratele and Shefer, 2002). Instead, the repeated representations of grief and guilt worked in Yoliswa's story against the lack of understanding and treatment shortage that had generated such unrepresentable grief and guilt. Yoliswa narrated her guilt both as entirely individual and inaccessible, and as a consequence of the sociomoral assault of treatment withholding. In that second narration, HIV moved away from abjection; the emotion of guilt became a political product.

If difficult emotions cannot always be made sense of in stories, it seems that in the genre of intimate disclosure at least they can make an appearance. Perhaps this is not surprising, since disclosure is never a complete or un-problematic event, but always a process, traversing uncertainties that can include emotional doubt and excess.

Other stories: the limits and possibilities of intimate disclosure as HIV ownership

Stories about 'coming to terms' with HIV have different emphases, depending on how the condition is lived in its specific social and historical location. In the UK by the late 1990s, stories of HIV support focused much more on individual acceptance, less on speaking out, and often ended up 'backgrounding' HIV into one of many life factors, important, chronic but controllable (Squire, 2006). Retrospective accounts of early stages of the epidemic were, however, more concerned with building HIV community, as with these South African interviewees.

In the South African context of a general policy and popular silence around HIV until around 2000, 'speaking out' appeared to have a significance con-nected with 'owning' the virus: believing in and accepting it, living positively with it, and becoming an active, speaking citizen of an HIV 'community' that takes in the whole nation. In talking to us, interviewees were expanding their HIV 'communities' of talk, and theorising how to do this further. These were processes they were engaged in regardless of the research. They were already looking for, and increasingly, finding, audiences ready to hear about HIV, and telling intimate disclosure stories that theorised previous steps along the path in order to take the next one.

The heterogeneity and fractures within genres mean that they undermine themselves constantly (Derrida, 1992). When analysing genres, we wouldn't expect stories to be perfect cases of, for instance, intimate disclosure. This qualification in our expectations about genres is valuable when looking at people's representations of ambiguous emotions around HIV. It encourages us to view people's strategies for addressing HIV as fluid, their use of one story genre as connected to others. While intimate disclosure narratives promoted 'ownership' of the virus and built HIV knowledge, understanding and action, such stories were not always appropriate or effective. Moreover, while speaking out, 'talking only', is an important pragmatic way of negotiating and theorising HIV, other stories also get told that help conduct people through their lives with HIV. These other genres are the focus of the next chapters.

5 Living positively

Religious and moral narratives of HIV[1]

AIDS has 'come to assume all the features of a traditional morality play: images of cancer and death, or blood and semen, of sex and drugs, or morality and retribution. A whole gallery of folk devils have been introduced – the sex-crazed gay, the dirty drug abuser, the filthy whore, the blood-drinking voodoo-driven black – side by side with a gallery of 'innocents' – the haemophiliacs, the blood transfusion 'victim', the new-born child, even the 'heterosexual'.

Kenneth Plummer, 1995: 177–8

I think stigma has been the priority for the churches because it decimates families, and people are not able to test themselves because of the stigma, and also I think the church has peddled a false theology of saying that if you are affected with HIV and AIDS you must have done something wrong, and therefore we are preaching a gospel which says, HIV and AIDS is not a punishment from God, it is a disease that is treatable, that is manageable and that can be prevented.

Archbishop Njongonkulu Ndungane, 2005

So what I want, like I am interested in other people, understand who are like me, like counselling people, understand. To clarify as in, okay, if one has HIV like what kind of a person are you, how do you live like something like that, understand. Like, I have tried it, understand I have talked to many people, like trying to explain like what happens, for instance there is a woman that came to the clinic while I was there. This woman, she came and I could see shame she was thinking a lot, this thing was very deep in her heart. But I tried to explain to her that 'no man this is not the end of the journey, you know. God is able to give us more life, understand. So do not be like that, understand, it is the Devil that gave us these diseases, it is not God, you see'. So really this woman said 'no man brother I wish I could always be with you because why, you encouraged me in the sense that I feel strong with the words that you gave me, understand'. So I am saying that these are the things that we were told about before, that okay these things {diseases} will happen, you see, but we won't give up hope, we will always believe in God that he is alive, so he will cleanse us and rebuke all these things {diseases} that we have in life. So I am looking at reaching counselling and preaching to people, understand.

Vuyani, Khayelitsha, June 2001

Introduction

In April 2001, I was beginning research on HIV support, based in Cape Town. I got in touch with a few interviewees who travelled, in several buses or taxis, from townships to the leafy suburban campus, to sit in front of my tape recorder. These interviewees usually had little support for living with HIV. They believed and accepted their HIV positive status, but they knew few with whom they could talk about their status, even within their families, and sometimes belief and acceptance were hard to maintain.

At the end of April, myself and a research assistant arrive at a large township clinic which provides general medical care as well as TB, antenatal and HIV services. By 9am, the waiting rooms are full, the narrow corridors lined with people, doctors and nurses squeezing by on tiptoe. We go to the adjacent office of an NGO that provides HIV advice, a tiny room shared by a counsellor and social worker. People often burst in; patient confidentiality is hard to maintain. Paint is peeling and facilities are few, but patients with HIV can be counselled and if they are ill, referred to another NGO clinic that offers treatment. We spend the day talking to people who have found their way to these cutting-edge HIV services. Their acceptance of HIV seems, unsurprisingly, firmer than that of the previous interviewees, resting on the hopes provided by treatment possibilities but also on the medical and counselling communities of interpretive support to which they now belong. Very often, they say they want support with their HIV positive lives from support groups. They want to be part of an interpretive community of people like them, within which their HIV beliefs and acceptance can be affirmed.

The following week, myself and another research assistant interview some women who attend an MTCT support group. For nine months, the women meet fortnightly, for an hour, in groups of up to 20. From these interviewees, we hear that the groups saved them. In these groups, they are able to believe in and accept their HIV status fully, to hear from others that they are not alone, and that their problems can be overcome. The groups seem to be operating not just as interpretive communities but as faith communities, allowing the women collectively to construct an ethics of HIV life. Interviewees describe affirming their 'conversions' to HIV belief and acceptance, and going out from the groups to testify to others, telling them what HIV is really like and how to deal with it, almost like a religious mission.

This chapter charts contemporary religious responses to HIV in South Africa and their development since the mid-1990s. In particular, it examines the place of religion, and religious structures of representation, in our interviewees' talk about HIV.

My interest in genres of HIV storytelling started from the assumption that personal narratives and cultural narratives, like those rooted in religious traditions, are interconnected. This is not a new idea: it is self-evident that individuals tell their stories within the narrative structures of their cultures

(Malik, 2000; Plummer, 1995; Riessman, 1993). But it is important to frame this supposition in ways that are appropriate to the particular situation. The argument in Chapter 4, that 'speaking out' is a means to HIV citizenship, owes much to Plummer's (1995) writing on the significance of self-disclosure narratives in an age of 'intimate citizenship'. However, the chapter frames the argument within the specific circumstances of the South African 'epidemic' of HIV-related silence. This chapter makes a more direct comparison between personal and 'cultural' narratives. It focuses on the links between religious conversion narratives, identified, for instance, among US and UK evangelical protestants of the seventeenth centuries and today,[2] a host of associated cultural and literary products – and the stories our interviewees told about coming to terms with HIV. The chapter suggests that some of those stories could be understood as representing moral progressions towards 'open' and ethical forms of living with HIV – that is, as HIV 'conversion' narratives – as well as representing social progression towards knowledge, acceptance and action.

The 'conversion' genre was not the only religious or moral strategy used in people's HIV stories, but it was an obvious and important one. By transforming people with HIV into ethical speakers and subjects, it worked as a resistance to HIV's moral, behavioural and bodily stigmatisation. Our interviewees also seemed to use it as the basis for a general, non-denominational, ethical narration of how to live life with HIV.

The significance of religious discourse for HIV in South Africa

If you are going to make comparisons between specific cultural narratives and personal stories, there need to be some criteria for doing so.[3] My interest in how interviewees' stories drew on religious narratives came from a number of sources. First, myself and the research assistants recognised how often interviewees talked spontaneously about religion, and how central it was to their lives, either through personal belief and prayer, church attendance and worship, or both. Second, we were interested early on in the interviews' religious-sounding emphases on 'belief' in and 'acceptance' of HIV status, and interviewees' insistence on the importance of telling others, or testifying.[4] Third, biblical or religious-sounding forms of languages were notable in both English and Xhosa sections of interviews. While we could not judge whether research participants deployed this language with especially high frequency around HIV, since that was the principal topic we talked about with them, its prominence indicated the strong currency of such language for our interviewees. Fourth, interviewees very often advanced religious explanations of HIV, alongside their medical accounts. As we saw in Chapter 3, these explanations were diverse, but did not involve personal blame. They seemed rather to be attempts to make sense of the sudden calamity of the epidemic within a familiar and persuasive moral frame, demonstrating once more the significance for the interviewees of religious discourse. Fifth, the existing literature on conversion narratives within theology and literary studies described story structures moving through confessions of struggle and denial, through acceptance, coming into faith and continuing tests of faith, and into testifying (Hindmarsh, 2005; Shea, 1968; Stromberg, 1993). These paths bore a strong relation both to our interviewees' stories of moving from 'othering' to 'owning' HIV, and to more general accounts of intimate disclosure stories such as Plummer's (1995).

There were some more general reasons why religious structures of talk seemed as if they might relate importantly to talk about HIV. Religious discourse has a strong profile in South African politics, civil society and popular media that it does not have so widely, across classes, ethnicities and cultural backgrounds, in all other countries, particularly the developed-world countries where personal HIV narratives have mostly been studied. Even where religious discourse is socially and culturally prominent – elsewhere in the developing world; in many working class and ethnic minority communities in the developed world; and throughout the US, which continues to show the highest developed-world rates of regular religious observance (Inglehart and Norris, 2004) – such discourse rarely has the recent history of effective political resistance that accompanies it in South Africa. Here, the oppression of apartheid was often figured as spiritual, as well as political, social and economic. Bloke Modisane's poem, quoted at the beginning of Chapter 4, eloquently conveys this spiritual attrition, as well as the possibility of being heard. Churches sometimes operated in collaboration with or support of apartheid, and critiques of Christianity more generally have been integral to analyses of colonialism in Africa. However, the African National Congress was from its earliest days associ-ated with a scripturally-rooted resistance to injustice (Hastings, 1994; Mphaphlele, 1962: 62–3; Tambo, 1987: 186ff.). Apartheid was effectively countered not just politically and socially, but also by a version of liberation theology, drawing on the African–American struggle tradition of Martin Luther King and expressed most obviously to the developed world in the writings and speeches of Desmond Tutu (2006 [1989]). Njongonkulu Ndungane, the succeeding Anglican Archbishop of Cape Town, continues this radical vision in his formulation of Christianity as a struggle against poverty, an expression of faith close to South American liberation theology at the same time as it emphasises its African context (Pato, 1997; see also Koopman, 2005).

There are numerous everyday indicators of religion's continuing significance in South Africa: 56 per cent of the population regularly attend religious services (Inglehart and Norris, 2004), 80 per cent identify as Christian, often as members of African independent churches and increas-ingly as members of evangelical and charismatic congregations, and another

5 per cent identify with other religions. Faith tends to correlate with concern about poverty and mild social and political conservatism (Policy Coordination and Advisory Services, 2006). Religion is ubiquitous in popular culture. Women's magazines, for instance, include religious education as part of their menu of childrearing advice; talk shows deploy religious as well as psychological vocabularies. Observances of faith were clearly important for many interviewees, who spent large parts of Sunday in worship; some devoted other days in the week also to religious activities.

The significance of religious faith and institutions for HIV prevention and treatment is widely recognised in many high HIV-prevalence situations. Religion and spirituality have been shown, for instance, to promote HIV coping and even physiological health in African–American communities (Tarakeshwar *et al.*, 2006; Woods *et al.*, 1999). Religion's role is, though most widely acknowledged in sub-Saharan Africa (Mahlangu-Ngcobo, 2001), in organisations such as Churches United in the Struggle against HIV/AIDS in Southern and Eastern Africa.[7] Faith-based organisations provide important care and sometimes, prevention initiatives, across Africa in resource-limited communities with strong faith commitments (Rosenberg *et al.*, 2004). Religious denomination, and attendance at religious services, appears in South Africa and Malawi to relate to rate of HIV positivity and high HIV-risk practices – although it is hard to get reliable data on the latter (Trinatopoli and Regnerus, 2005). The political strengths of religious discourse and practice in South Africa, alongside the entire nation's high HIV prevalence, give it particular salience there.

HIV has, however, had a contested relation to religion across all countries and faiths affected by it. Plummer's description, quoted at the beginning of this chapter, of the condemning cultural 'morality plays' written about people with HIV, gives an apt summary of the widespread religiously inflected discourse of HIV stigma. In South Africa, as elsewhere on the continent (Iliffe, 2006: 94–7) this involved many initial characterisations of HIV as a gay, therefore western, disease and gay people as sinners, and of people with HIV as sexual transgressors – again, initially, as western, but later with women, as we saw in the previous chapter, strongly associated with the abjection of sexual rule-breaking. Condoms were figured as irreligious and perhaps themselves contaminated with HIV; abstinence as the only acceptable prevention method; and the virus itself as divine punishment. These characterisations significantly retarded HIV prevention and treatment. Even now, 'religiosity' can detract from HIV education's effectiveness when it restricts the communication of the 'life skills' curriculum in schools (Cherian, 2004). However, churches' approaches to the epidemic have shifted markedly. For instrumental as well as ethical reasons, most have adopted a more supportive role as the scale of the epidemic within their own congregations becomes apparent. Many are committed, sometimes problematically, to praying for improvement or even cure. Condoms are everywhere in church discourse, and even in 2001, for our most explicitly religious interviewees, impediments to condom use were social, not religious. Recognising the need for a more integrated and complex approach, the Uganda-based African Network of Religious Leaders Living with or personally affected by HIV/AIDS, working with Christian Aid, has moved from Abstain, Be faithful, Condomise, to a new SAVE model of HIV work: Safer practices, Available medications, Voluntary counselling and testing, Education.[8] Increasingly, churches mount practical efforts at support, prevention and education, and become involved in advocacy and activism. Traditional healing based on spiritual beliefs has similarly moved from characterising people with HIV as spiritual transgressors or the victims of spiritual transgressors, towards a less blame-orientated understanding.[9] Many faiths in South Africa, as in the rest of the world, have powerful communities of women within them (Gaitskell, 1997), and sectors that promote equal rights for gay men and lesbians, which also advocate for the rights of HIV positive people, and support-related campaigns against sexual abuse and violence.[10]

The church's status as a focus of political-ethical activism seems to have declined in the 'new' South Africa (Laubscher, 2003). Yet religious institutions could be said to be regaining their ethical focus through their HIV work. Religious and political leaders emphasise that living 'with' HIV, whatever one's status, is itself a religious act, a test of faith and charity. Archbishop Ndungane's address to HIV, for instance, focuses on opposing stigma and the 'false theology' of conceptualising HIV as punishment, and promoting programmes for prevention, treatment and 'loving care'. Ndungane was himself publicly tested at a free voluntary testing and counselling site in a township (Ndungane, 2005). Mandela – regarded as a major ethical figure by most South Africans – challenged religious stigma around HIV when he declared the disease which killed his son was not 'an illness reserved for people who are going to go to hell and not to heaven' (*New York Times*, 7 January 2005). At the commemoration service for Treatment Action Campaign activist Christopher Moraka, Reverend S. Mema of the Ethiopian Church of Southern Africa declared, 'none of us invites HIV into our bodies, so it is unacceptable to discriminate against those living with AIDS' (*City Vision*, 21 October 2004). This new Christian ethics of HIV-affected life has been taken up more generally. As a letter-writer to the South African women's magazine, *Soul*, puts it in describing her relation to an HIV positive friend:

> I was so happy that one of my friends disclosed her status to me immediately after testing positive and as a child of God I was there to counsel and tell her how much God loves her. And HIV/AIDS is not the end of the world. Actually it is the beginning of a new journey with God. ... Let us support people who are HIV positive and love them like before we knew their status. Some of the people who are not supporting them

are positive themselves so go and have a test today and begin another journey with Jesus and don't give the devil a chance to rejoice.[11]

Religious discourse has thus, like South African HIV talk in general, moved from 'othering' to 'owning' the virus. As we saw in preceding chapters, however, this move has not necessarily translated into acceptance and openness for individual members of faith communities. Moreover, speaking about HIV still involves speaking against the powerful earlier religious story of HIV as the outcome, sign or stigma of immorality or wrongdoing. For the Greeks, a stigma was a mark *imposed* on the morally defective; for Christians it *arose* on the morally good or the physically disordered. The extended application of the term 'stigma' to non-obvious undesired or 'discreditable' (Goffman, 1963) conditions such as HIV works, alongside the Christian version, because we hold onto a version of the Greek negative moral significance of imposed stigma. Moral defectiveness is seen as being played out through discredited and discreditable conditions. Occasionally this gets reversed, in for instance the secular and sometimes religious canonisation of suffering. Some images of HIV – for example the Benetton advertisement, 'The Pièta', showing dying AIDS activist David Kirby on a hospital bed surrounded by grieving family (Toscano, 2002) – have displayed this 'positive' version of HIV stigma. However, the condition's powerful associations with states close to what Kristeva (1984) calls the abjection of sexual and social rule-breaking, illness and death have generated almost uniformly negative stigmatisations, rendering it trangressive even to talk about (Dowling, n.d.). To speak openly about HIV, owning it, as our interviewees did, is therefore to speak against this persisting morality tale of HIV as transgression and abjection, and to try, like the letter-writer above, to tell a new one.

HIV 'conversion' narratives

As an example, I want to return to our interview with Linda, one of the women who was participating in support groups as part of an MTCT programme. In Chapter 3, I quoted Linda's account of how she talked to her reluctant, disbelieving husband continually about HIV. Eventually, he came to believe and accept her positive status, and to support her. In Chapter 4, we saw this extract in its larger narrative context, bracketed by Linda's story of her own HIV acceptance, her earlier participation in the 'interpretive community' of a support group, and her plans to be more open about her status. In Chapter 4 though, I omitted a small section of Linda's story – just four sentences at the end, where Linda describes how religion has inflected her approach to HIV. This section acts retrospectively to put the whole story into a narrative frame informed by religion. Here, again, is Linda's account of coming to accept her HIV status, recapitulated from Chapter 4, but also including her account of the virus's relation to religion:

Linda: Okay! In the first place I am glad that I know of my HIV positive status because now I know what to do. Then my husband, the one I am married to, I told him. At first, he could not accept it, he gave me too many problems. I then continued talking about it everyday, I used to chat about it so that it would sink into him that I am a person who is HIV positive. /mhm/ Truly, eventually he accepted it. It was before my baby was not discharged yet, so that /he could be tested as well. /okay!/ Then he asked about the baby. I said the baby will be tested at nine months. I then explained. Truly then I was told that the baby, I was very happy, because I was happy to save my baby. AZT helped me, my baby was tested negative. That made me a very happy person, I didn't think of myself as having HIV because I am still alright. There is no difference I must say. My health is still good. The other thing that made me happy is the group support that we are doing as nursing mothers. /mhm/ It really really helped us because you feel free when you are there I must say. You become very happy and forget that eish, when you get home it is then that you remember that you have HIV, but when you are there you are free. We advise each other very well, even the instructor {facilitator}, I must say she tells us what to do, so today I am not ready, I am not yet free, I don't feel like I am open, I am not open yet to stand up and say I have HIV. I will keep trying, you understand? /Mhm/ But I feel alright, most importantly I thank God. God said these things before, he said there will be these incurable diseases, so I believe in God truly. What he talked about, is happening today. So that is something else that inspired me, because God mentioned this before, he said they will happen, they are happening today, unto people, they would not fall in steep places, so I believe in that.

This is a story of HIV support, as described in Chapter 3 – including the ethical support offered by a religious explanation of the epidemic: 'he said there will be these incurable diseases' – and a story of interpretive community, as explored in Chapter 4. Yet the story also exemplifies a religious storytelling genre on which many interviewees drew to structure their stories of HIV. In these stories, 'seroconversion' is followed by a 'conversion' to HIV belief, knowledge and acceptance. An HIV positive identity becomes a religious or at least a moral one. Research participants described a struggle to confront HIV status, culminating in a mental and emotional 'conversion', marked in the stories by people saying something like, 'then, I believed', or – as here – 'eventually he accepted it'. Such an acceptance or conversion moment might come before the test; after the test, in post-test counselling; some time later; or even, as with Michael, after three illnesses, three HIV tests, and after his girlfriend biblically asked him 'three times' about the results of his final test, impelling him to tell her and no longer 'hide it'.

For women like Linda, who were participating in MTCT programmes, the 'conversion' moment of acceptance was frequently revisited in the salvational event of their baby testing negative, a deliverance ineluctably linked in the stories to the availability of medication: 'truly then I was told that the baby, I was very happy because I was happy to save my baby. AZT helped me'. However, as in many religious narratives, there were ongoing doubts on the long and difficult path towards faith – in this case, HIV knowledge and belief. This is a problematic journey of improvement: 'I will keep still trying, understand?', Linda says. Such ambiguities are part of the generic structure of conversion narratives, but they are not always easily manageable within it. Theologians have long expressed concerns about the tensions in conversion narratives between formula and idiosyncrasy, individualism and the common experience of faith, continuity and division between the past and the present (Jacobs, 2003; Shea, 1968). 'Conversion' stories of coming to terms with HIV are, though, new, diverse and difficult enough to navigate the ambiguities of HIV 'acceptance' without becoming formulaic.

The trope of active, even welcoming acceptance in the stories, indicates how interviewees formulated their lives with the virus as a 'conversion' of HIV itself. The virus can be 'converted' into something bearable, even godly, by the way it is lived with. Sipho called his status God's will, but this will is not a revengeful one, and he relied on God's voice to help him and his wife, rather than conflating HIV with the sin of blame:

> **Sipho**: I just came to terms with the situation and told myself that pointing fingers was not going to sort things out. We just needed to fix our ears unto God and told ourselves that what had happened was due to God's will.

The conversion moment was thus for Sipho and others, as is apparent too in other places in the pandemic (Squire, 2006), a moment not just of acceptance but also of taking on HIV as a spiritual task, with the implication that God judges you strong enough to bear it. It might mean changing your life in concrete ways, moving away from old friends who do not understand HIV or who live unethically in relation to the virus. Men like Vuyani said they used to have many girlfriends but now had found God within their newly ethical HIV positive lives and relationships. Some women said they now spent more time in church as part of their programme of caring for their HIV positive bodies and minds, less time out socialising and drinking.

Many interviewees told of searching out HIV versions of faith communities to strengthen their beliefs – places where they, like Linda, could be open and even cheerful about their status. As we saw earlier, support groups often provided this when family and friendship groups did not. Here, HIV status could and indeed must be confessed, and one could be reborn as a person living positively with HIV, in a kind of secular 'grace':

knowing how to eat, exercise, prevent transmission and get treatment, and looking forward to a long and healthy life. Talk in the groups set people 'free', as Linda described. It provided an almost biblical transformation, achieved by knowing – and, indissolubly connected to this, speaking of – HIV's truths.[12] The evils of HIV and its attendant anxieties were narrated as lifted by open confession and testimony. Sylvia, for instance, told how a nurse asked who she could talk to and declared that such talk would allow her HIV troubles – like the 'thorn in the flesh', the satanic demon troubling St Paul – to 'depart from' her.[13]

Participants' stories often extended this liberatory openness to describe a wider HIV 'witnessing', something like an evangelical mission, aimed at converting others to the speaker's own accepting, knowledgeable and ethical life with HIV. Chapter 4 contained many examples of this broader speaking out, without examining its links to religious discourse. As we saw there, telling your status to your partner and family was usually the first step in giving HIV testimony, as for Linda with her husband; but witnessing could spread much wider. Like testifying to faith, living openly with HIV becomes a kind of spiritual mission or destiny, a way of 'doing God's work', as Gilbert and Wright (2002: 34; 139ff.) describe hearing within the stories of HIV positive African–American women. Busisiwe's concern to talk about HIV to family, friends, young people and even go on television is a good example. Busisiwe explicitly presents this desire as originating in church and moving outwards:

> **Busisiwe**: Church is very important because I can't stay there and say 'please God help me'. I need just three years to live so as to tell people about HIV, and I'll try with my friends.[14]

At times, such witnessing was done, as we saw in Chapters 3 and 4, through a kind of 'non-disclosing acceptance'. The importance of healthy, 'positive' living with HIV was promulgated in general terms, without the evangelical power of first-person testifying. Stories like these were for some interviewees, as they still are for many in South Africa, an important moral step along the route to 'openness' and 'freedom'. But South Africa's history of the moral vilifying of positive people, meant that personal testimony of being yourself HIV positive, driven by a kind of 'priesthood of the believer', was many interviewees' ethical as well as social goal. Elsewhere in her interview, Linda – talking after her support group acquaintance Phumla had described the importance of going out and helping people – specified the place of personal disclosure, giving 'personal testimony' in this process, 'so that the weak can become stronger and learn from you that you are also strong'.

Linda's longer story of HIV acceptance, struggle, faith and testimony becomes clearly entwined with Christian discourse at its end. It seems to reference Psalm 91's account of 'noisome pestilence' and God's protection of the faith from it: 'no evil (shall) befall thee, neither shall any plague come nigh thy dwelling'. It does not reference this text literally, as meaning that faith will entirely shield one from or cure HIV, but rather as making it possible to live with it. It also seems in Linda's last sentence that she is invoking Isaiah, a book frequently used by religious speakers and writers in addressing HIV, and, before that, apartheid, civil rights struggles and slavery. Isaiah prophecies the punishment of the wicked, the protection of the faithful, and in this story, the road being made clear through the wilderness of this new condition of HIV to the city of God – the right way of living with the condition: 'Every valley shall be exalted, and every mountain and hill shall be made low: and the crooked shall be made straight, and the rough places plain.'[15]

Like Linda, describing her process of coming to terms with HIV, many interviewees used elements of religious language in allusive and illuminating ways, perhaps particularly in relation to this topic. Another common association, for instance, seemed to be with Psalm 37's assertion of God's support for the good, poor and faithful in times of difficulty and wickedness, with 'wickedness' connoting inhuman reactions to the epidemic rather than HIV status or behaviours related to it. Listeners like me, relatively unfamiliar with religious languages as well as, in this case, the interview language itself, may miss many of these moral reframings and reclaimings of HIV, which are likely to characterise talk about the virus in many other high-prevalence contexts where religious faith is central to people's lives.[16]

Despite the explicit Christian references at the end of Linda's story, perhaps more persuasive evidence of its link to the conversion genre was the way in which it was followed up by Linda's cointerviewee, Lindi, an acquaintance from her support group. As if she is indeed in the HIV faith community of the support group rather than an interview, Lindi follows Linda's testimony with the story of her own 'conversion': her path towards openness about HIV. Like Linda's, this is a story of 'conversion' to moral HIV subjecthood: 'I do not criticise myself any more, I am the same as other people'.

> **Lindi**: Okay. The first time I heard was last year in July /mhm/ I took a very long time, thinking about this, thinking about who am I going to tell first, what am I going to do. I gave birth in October, and also in October I also joined the support group, here. And then after being involved in the support group, I then could plan, I wrote a list, writing people's names that I could tell. At first on the list it was my mother, but I haven't told her because I am still scared. The second one was my boyfriend, I haven't told him yet as well, the third was my sister all three of them I wrote them in the book. Ever since I joined the support group, I don't want to lie, it helped me the most. I do not tell {criticise} myself any more, because I learnt that I am the same as other people, I live just like them. The only reason that would make me tell them, what would make me happy is if my baby can be tested negative. I feel like I would be motivated and encouraged to tell them that I am HIV positive but the baby has nothing.

For Lindi, then, like Linda, HIV acceptance is a process, and the HIV status of her baby could be salvational. The support group acts as a faith community, and generates plans for further testimonies, particularly to close family and friends, which are steps on the path towards openness and truth. Linda's own account of her plans for community work, coming just after Phumla's rather similar story of her projected home care and educational work, constitutes a further example of such chains of testimony. Joint interviews' sequences of similar personal stories might be regarded in conventional research terms as exhibiting social coercion and neglecting the individual significances of HIV. However, I think they can be understood better here as examples of the powerful modality of collective, ethical testimony.

At times, HIV 'conversion' stories were also told in relation to non-Christian traditional spiritual beliefs, again with a structure moving towards enlightenment and its spread. Busisiwe, for instance, after the birth of her stillborn baby, had dreams about her ancestors that led to her acceptance of HIV, as we saw in Chapter 4. Her account of these dreams was also followed by stories of her desire to use her power – which comes from God and must be used 'as when one is preaching' to find out more about HIV and to tell her friends and everyone else about the condition:

> **Busisiwe**: So, I do (really) value that they {ancestors} give me brightness and drive away darkness. What I want now is to be shown things {about how to treat and/or cure HIV} . . . there is a need for a better treatment to be added or found. God can choose one person to explain the ingredients of the cure which is what I want . . . I have a sense of humour like the other lady {in the support group} who was joking about this. I realised that I could do it too. I can joke about it until a person understands it. So, people would see that I also have this and that I'm free and not anxious. . . . This must be done in a free spirit as one becomes free when s/he is preaching in the church hoping even that his/her prayer is ascending.

Here a narrative of conversion and witnessing, rooted in the 'free spirit' of faith, unproblematically brings together Christianity and traditional beliefs. Many South African healers similarly hold these two belief systems in parallel (Peltzer *et al.*, 2006), despite their formal incommensurability within the evangelical Christianity espoused by a number of our interviewees.

Secular conversions

Research participants like Lindi drew on a religious genre of conversion and witnessing which was structural, not marked by explicit talk about religion, but still moving, with difficulty and self-reflection, from conflict to conversion.[17] Like the more obviously 'religious' stories, these narratives too mapped out a path towards ethical living with HIV. It was this trajectory towards morally correct living, as much as religious resonances of form, language and subjecthood, that made conversion narratives effective in the interviews and perhaps outside them. Interwoven with interviewees' stories of socially owning the virus and speaking out about it, these conversion pathways mapped out difficult but achievable journeys towards ethical citizenship with HIV.

Acceptance, knowledge and testimony were, as Chapter 4 showed, so prominent a focus of people's stories that they seemed at times like imperatives. They were tied to a kind of life discipline that, while it has clear health significance, is also an ethical, but not a specifically religious requirement: the requirement to live the right kind of life. Mhiki, as we saw in Chapter 3, made acceptance the prerequisite for ethical HIV life: 'With regard to things that are helpful to one who is living with HIV firstly, you must accept it.' Vuyani similarly related his acceptance, and that of others, to a sense of ethical life that goes beyond specifically religious reference, as the quotation at the beginning of the chapter demonstrates. Vuyani accepts and brings others to acceptance through his formulation of HIV positive life in a religious frame – 'God is able to give us more life, understand' – and he wants to witness to his HIV understanding in a way that combines religion with education and therapy: 'I am looking at teaching, counselling and preaching to people.' But the overall goal he sets up at the beginning of this story is the elucidation of an ethical rather than a religious subject of HIV: 'if one has HIV . . . what kind of a person are you, how do you live'. I shall return to this broader, pragmatic narrative of ethical living, at once secular *and* religious, later in the chapter. First, it is important to look at the limitations conversion narratives come up against in representing HIV.

The limits of conversion

A genre's imperfections mean, as we saw in the previous chapter, that aspects of people's lives that are hard to make sense of within 'stories' as they are conventionally understood, can still appear within a 'genre'. The genre continues, imperfectly, around them. Crises of HIV 'faith', for instance, could appear in Linda's narrative of immanent, not-yet-achieved belief. She is ready but also not ready to speak of HIV; she is on the interminable road to community and faith that conversion narratives map out. Lindi too has planned to speak out about HIV, but she has not yet done so; Busisiwe and Vuyani have discussed their status, though not as widely as they would like. Some things that cannot be said at all – about grief and guilt, for instance – can be left as a speaking silence. Within religious conversion narratives such struggle is, arguably, so standardised a feature that it lacks the power to challenge or change mainstream representations. Translated into the novel and less conventionalised field of talk about HIV, conversion narratives' contemporary ability to include ambiguities, allows personal and political difficulties that are crucial to understanding and living HIV positive lives, to appear within the stories.

It is possible that even when conversion narratives address the different field of HIV 'faith' in apparently secular ways, they retain elements of regulation derived from their religious beginnings. Perhaps you have to be religious, at least at the level of culture, to use the lexicon of belief, testimony and ethical living that makes you part of even a secular HIV 'faith community'. Perhaps secular conversion narratives are always implicitly religious. 'Acceptance', for instance, though never fully attainable, was, as we have seen, an imperative, and involved an agentic Christian welcoming of HIV as a kind of guest – albeit of the uninvited variety, as Reverend S. Mema pointed out. It seemed at times to mark a religiously shaded ethical imperative. HIV 'belief', a word with strong religious connotations, was a close accompaniment to acceptance. These linkages can at times promote an alternative discourse of HIV transgression, pointing at those who do not 'accept' the virus as betraying the new ethico-religious project around HIV. Perhaps, too, religiously defined 'transgressions' around sexuality are again rendered unspeakable within HIV versions of conversion narratives. Such prescriptiveness is at present, however, a minor concern. These secularised 'conversion' narratives are so broadly formulated around HIV, they seem largely to avoid becoming regulatory ethics.

We might, finally, ask whether the resonance of people's stories with religious genres of discourse really matters much; after all, it's just talk. As Stromberg (1993) and Mbembe (2001) point out, however, conversion is a linguistic act. It depends precisely on the conversion *narrative*, on having and speaking the true language. Saying of HIV, 'I have it', is not just a phrase, but a no-going-back act. Similarly, a 'conversion story' of the right way to understand and live with HIV, when the condition has previously been silenced or recounted as a transgression, is a social as well as a linguistic practice. It demonstrates the ethics of the speaker's HIV-positive life, as well as simply representing that life.

Following Plummer (1995), who relates interpretive communities to communities of action, I am assuming that the interconnection between conversion genre and personal HIV narratives can potentiate personal narratives' effects. The conversion genre was recognisable to our interviewees, ourselves and wider South African speech communities. It worked to turn stories of HIV into morality tales. Our interviewees' stories borrowed the ethical force of the conversion genre and gave it to living with HIV, previously the object of some quite different religious stories. Their stories of their lives became morality tales about how one ought to live with the condition. This HIV conversion genre does not simply produce reversals, but rather a kind of double vision, a doubled sense of the world before and after this new story. It relates, liminally, to the processes that are always occurring on the abject edges of faith 'community', making its boundaries uncertain.

For women in particular, to tell such stories was to speak back to religious discourse, not rejecting it, but using it to claim their status as moral, not abjected, subjects.

The conversion genre was a powerful one at this specific time and place. But it might also occur in other situations where people are trying to formulate stories of self and community, against their pathologisation and marginalisation. What Goffman (1963: 37) calls 'exemplary moral tales' often arise among groups of stigmatised people. Norman Denzin (1993) has described a conversion, through spoken and other interactions, to shared 'alcoholic' identities within Alcoholics Anonymous 12-step programmes that are explicitly modelled on religious faith. 'Coming out' stories of lesbian and gay sexuality in the UK and US draw on the liberating power of conversion stories (Plummer, 1995). Like religious South African HIV stories, they reclaim the resonance of a religious plot previously used to exclude their tellers from moral subjecthood. The telling of morality tales about coming to terms with and living with HIV, however, has a different span of potential effects. High-prevalence countries are also often highly religiously observant, with a history of condemnatory religious stories about HIV. The assumption of moral HIV subjecthood through HIV 'conversion' narratives might work to establish social and political citizenship generally in such contexts, not just in South Africa.

Ethical living with HIV

As we have seen, interviewees often told secularised versions of HIV 'conversion' narratives that made them into broadly ethical rather than religious progressions. I want now to look at how our research participants presented their lives with HIV more widely as ethical projects of self-cultivation. These projects, like the traditions of 'care of the self' described by Foucault (1988), drew on religious discourses and practices, but were also to an important degree autonomous of them, operating pragmatically within the new field of HIV life to knit historically and socially distinct ethical patterns into contemporary alliance.

Conventional religions' ambiguity about HIV is one factor supporting such secularisation of HIV ethics. Another is the necessity of doctrinal openness in ethical thinking in South Africa, in order to address not just Christianity, but traditional African belief systems, Islam, Hinduism and Judaism. This openness is, indeed, constitutionally guaranteed. Moreover, as Mkhise (2004) notes, there is a long history of traditional spiritualities' coexistence with Christianity, in South Africa as in many other developing-world countries, producing specific forms of Christianity (Oosthuisen and Hexham, 1989; Pretorius and Jafta, 1997) and inflecting conventional Christian denominations. The ANC was, as Oliver Tambo noted, the 'virtual incubator' of ecumenism in South Africa (1987: 188). The framing of both organised religious and 'spiritual' life practices in the unifying terms of subjective experience seems increasingly significant in South Africa, as in other contexts (Heelas and Woodhead, 2005). In *AIDS in Africa: An African and Prophetic Perspective*, Mankekolo Mahlangu-Ngcobo, a South African-origin preacher exiled in the 1980s, considers Islam and ancestor beliefs alongside Christianity in analysing how religions must address HIV. She ends the book with a highly contextualised, practical prayer, calling for God to care for nurses and doctors, traditional healers, HIV educators and governments involved in the epidemic, and spiritually to 'heal' drug companies and international aid organisations, as well as African people themselves (2001: 57–60). Like Mahlangu-Ngcobo, people in South Africa, and elsewhere in the pandemic, tell stories about how to live with HIV within a number of political, personal, social and medical narrative frames, as well as those of conventional religions, that lead to a heterogeneous, ecumenical perspective on ethical HIV lives.

The correct ways of living with HIV of which people speak thus bring together different ethical narratives. For example, Vuyani follows the account of his ethical life quoted at the start of this chapter, which weaves together examination of the self and Christian faith, with a description of how he is also physically, psychologically and socially 'beautiful':

> **Vuyani**: Most people cannot believe when I tell them that no I have HIV. They would say 'hayi bo, but you look', I am beautiful, I look beautiful, I look healthy. I say 'no do not have this mindset that if you want to see an HIV positive person, you will see a sick person, understand, you will see someone who can't do anything. So a person lives with HIV in his/her body, but if he/she is disciplined, like {using} a condom, understand, {s/he will be ok}.'

It seemed that part of this new HIV ethics was to accept the limitations of human agency – an important rhetorical move, since the taking on of individual responsibility for health can be depressing and guilt-provoking when physical realities overwhelm it. This acceptance of limits was itself articulated both religiously and secularly. Something beyond personal agency decrees when you die, within traditional beliefs (Selikow *et al.*, 2002). External causation works similarly in Christianity, where death comes always as 'God's will'; and within medical, social and political understandings of HIV. When interviewees said that they might die any time, regardless of HIV, or that death comes to us all, or that we all die at our appointed time, such abnegations of individual agency brought together spiritual submission, with medical and political assessments of risk. Statistically, as people in South Africa are aware, there are high-frequency threats to longevity that rival HIV, such as non-HIV related TB, early childhood illnesses, and in middle age, conditions such as diabetes and heart disease, all of which are undertreated in resource-poor circumstances. People in the UK living with HIV similarly talk about the risks of death run by all of us; these are, however, generally conceptualised as accident and long-term health risks.

Such multiple formulations of HIV ethics and their limits were tied together in the interviews by general accounts of the right path in HIV life. Interviewees focused on how to care for the body, think about HIV, talk about HIV, act in sexual relationships, plan for your death and funeral, and provide for your family after death. Segments of this path were described in the stories of how to live positively with HIV that appeared in previous chapters. Across its whole span, such a narrative path constitutes a new genre of exemplary HIV life story, related to but not determined by religious narratives, a kind of everyday theory of ethical living of the kind Foucault (1988) describes. When interviewees talked of themselves as living a disciplined or correct life, they were indeed demonstrating this ethical life, within the microcommunity of the research structure. Speaking of ethical HIV life more generally, within the broader communities of 'loving care' that Ndungane calls for at this beginning of this chapter, such as family and friendship groups, was another way of realising it. Accepting, open, knowledgeable and forward-looking talk about HIV is both part of ethical HIV living, and a symbolisation of it.

However, the genre must be lived out, as well as spoken, and how you live your life also represents HIV ethics. For many interviewees who made only brief references to living correctly, these references appeared to index extensive performance of practices that need not be enumerated, since they belonged to a commonly held repertoire of good living, now invoked in the context of HIV, but of older and more wide-ranging provenance (Holdstock, 2000).

Self-government is a Christian imperative with a particularly strong protestant cast, but with wider religious and non-religious antecedents. Today, it also constitutes a subject which is ideal ground for more psychological discourses. HIV ethics is, like other ethical programmes across the world, increasingly articulated around what Foucault called a 'conversion to the self', taking a psychological rather than a religious tone. For Michael, for instance, knowing about HIV is an ethical matter related to personal knowledge and growth that develops out of his religious faith:

> **Michael**: God has made that Michael can, you might know yourself you HIV positive so that you can do things and protect yourself and involve yourself to the HIV/AIDS activities /mhm/ and you know all those things, I always thank God, to know myself, in time that I'm HIV positive, so that I can do things properly.

If Augustine's confessions were about understanding the self through conversion, then the conversion narratives of the seventeenth century and later were more contradictorily involved with the speaking or writing of the self, at the same time as abnegating it. By the time of Rousseau's more secular *Confessions*, the self becomes, explicitly, a writer. For Rousseau, the self, not the truth, is the project (Stromberg, 1993). Rousseau plays with the impossibility of the self's complete conversion, of confessing all. In later 'confessional' writing (De Man, 1983) representation's own impossibilities are the subject. In describing a new HIV ethics through the self, another project makes itself evident: that of strategically establishing an HIV self and language, however contradictory and impossible, against their exclusion or abjectification in modern and postmodern conditions of representation and existence.[18]

Despite the new HIV ethics' psychological shading, religious discourse continues powerfully to shape it. The ethics' emphasis on mental and physical discipline comes from religious rules, even when its content does not. The idea of a code of responsible, right moral conduct is present both in the religious texts that many South Africans follow, and in older spiritual traditions in which one has to behave well in order to become a recognised adult person. Being recognised as 'a person among others', as Busisiwe describes it, in the manner of your life, death and mourning, is a matter of spiritual, not just social and personal, importance. Many interviewees were concerned that their stigmatised illness, alongside a poverty exacerbated by HIV, would deliver them to a meagre, sparsely attended, *inhuman* funeral, of which, as Zola put it, 'you can cry and say, "even a dog is not buried like this"'. The call to be recognised, living and dying, as 'a person' also draws on the symbolic resource of equality in faith current in religious discourse. This equality, spiritual but also political, was the endpoint of many interviewees' 'conversion' narratives of coming to terms with and talking openly about HIV.

As we have seen, the end is never really the end in such stories. The messaianic imagining of continual improvement in one's relation to HIV is also part of them. This teleology, always building towards a better ethical future, draws strongly on religious discourse. However, as is characteristic of pragmatism (West, 1989), our interviewees grounded these ethics of the future in the practicalities of what could be done. Pam, for instance, asked God to allow long enough for her, by her own actions, to safeguard her daughter's future, up to the age of 18. Religion provides the frame for her ethical imagining of the future, but this imagining is worked out within social constraints on health and education:

> **Pam**: The diet is changed /really/ because I want to live a long time because my firstborn is eight years and she's doing Grade Three /oh yeah/ at least, I want to survive for, a long time, at least when she's in tertiary level then I, then I can go to the grave /mhm/ I don't mind as long as she's an adult /mhm/ that's my wish /mhm/ I wish God /mhm/ can do that for me.

West (1989: 233) suggests that 'prophetic' pragmatism, a religiously based 'urgent and compassionate critique' rooted in Judeo-Christian traditions but more specifically, for him, in the African–American church, is the discourse that, in the US at least, most effectively ties oppositional criticism of the past to a progressive quest for the future. In South Africa, the insistent effects of religious discourse in talk about HIV reinstate people with HIV as moral subjects, and contribute to the construction of a new HIV life ethics. They serve to maintain the value of spirituality in relation to HIV, in the shape of a broadly formulated, non-prescriptive commitment to 'loving care' – the 'compassion' to which West refers. And they enable a path towards an enlightened, practical HIV future based on the struggles of the past.

To exemplify this new spiritual ethics of HIV life, deploying traditional religious genres in changed conditions, I want to recapitulate Busisiwe's formulations of her programme of HIV acceptance and communication. One of Busisiwe's most marked negotiations of this programme is in the area of sexual ethics. Ethics are, for writers such as Foucault and (differently) for Kristeva, fundamentally sexually regulatory, a character strengthened by their close relations with religious laws. Codifications of HIV sexual ethics can certainly be prescriptive. In the South African context, HIV guidelines from international NGOs are, as we have seen, often viewed as postcolonial attempts to exoticise and control African sexualities. However, in Busisiwe's account we see a witnessing to these new codes that allows her own negotiation of them, as she describes taking HIV sex education out from the clinic to her friends, and to her boyfriend, who responds to her testimony by calling for 'a whole plastic {bag} full of condoms, then I was thrilled'.

Christianity itself can be translated, for Busisiwe through popular culture especially, in order to pursue the new ethical project of HIV education and acceptance. She talks about the divine provenance of HIV hopes and possibility, and the importance of testifying to others about HIV. She also talks a great deal about popular culture as an ethical HIV medium. Here, she discusses books and *Soul City* magazines and programmes, and from this moves on to the power of gospel music as a counter to condemnations of the HIV positive:

> **Busisiwe**: So, sometimes you must take a book and see and read it, I'm not suggesting that you should study it but you can read *Soul City*'s magazines. *Soul City* has some lessons and sometimes I listen or and watch this programme. It is encouraging, because you love to see it on TV . . . {and I would like} for instance to sing. You see my sister I really enjoy gospel music like that of Rebecca {Malope}. Even if people are saying we are HIV positive, I just sing.

Finally, Busiswe demonstrates how traditional spirituality can be brought into contemporary HIV ethics, in her synthesising narratives of traditional beliefs, church and clinic, all in pursuit of better living and a cure. She says that prayer gives her strength: 'Most importantly it's God's word that I'm thirsty for, I don't want to lie about that . . . There is nothing that can overpower prayer.' She believes her power to discover a traditional solution through traditional means will be given by God. She also makes some creative appropriations of indigenous spirituality. For instance, she claims validation for her hopes of divination from Nongqause, the nineteenth-century girl who was, she says, 'gifted' with 'visions'. Nongqause's flawed vision of how to escape white occupation and oppression drove the Xhosa to kill their cattle and destroy their crops (Peires, 1989). But Busisiwe used her name to call up the power of Xhosa spirituality, particularly its foresight: a strong, ethically grounded knowledge that can be drawn on in the struggle with HIV.[19]

6 Talking politics

I would have hoped . . . that we would invoke the same spirit, the same passion, the same commitment to fight this pandemic as we had when we were fighting against the scourge of apartheid.

Desmond Tutu, 24 March 2002, SABC

Treatment activism teaches us that prevention is political. HIV prevention advocacy and activism must be placed on the agenda of every scientist, health professional, activist and community leader. HIV prevention advocacy must be scientifically rigorous. It must unequivocally defend the autonomy, dignity and equality of women and girl-children. It must promote the needs and protect the marginalized and vulnerable in every context, whether gay men, sex workers, injecting drug users, prisoners, migrants, refugees or children.

Zackie Achmat, 2006

Now that I'm HIV positive I don't feel different to the people who are not. No I'm a human being just like them. Yes I am HIV positive but they also have their sicknesses too /Sure, sure/ Of course they are not different with me, you see. So I take myself as a normal person just like anybody, you see. Of course I'm a normal person, you see. Yes, I am. So I don't I don't see them different to me, no, they are not. I still have rights just like them.

David, June 2001, Khayelitsha

Introduction

After several telephone calls and a preliminary chat with the coordinator, I meet with an HIV-focused community-based organisation (CBO) to see if some of its members would like to participate in our HIV support research. A group of around ten support group coordinators, mostly women, has assembled, along with the paid workers for the organisation, for their regular weekly meeting. The group asks me to describe the research, and I do so, handing out the leaflet about it that will be made available to participants. People read it carefully and ask questions about what will happen to the research and whether I will be making any money from it. One person suggests that an appropriate interviewee fee would be that paid to a lecturer or public speaker – around R350 a person. I say that I cannot afford this amount, that the R50 fee is based on the University of Cape Town research assistant scale, and that the research nature of the interview means that I will be talking to a lot of people, all of whom will be represented anonymously in the study reports, so the interviewees will not be in the position of public speakers. Some people seem okay with this. I get the impression from others that they do not see a great difference between the appropriations of experience and knowledge that happen in radio and television broadcasting, and those that happen in research. In the 2001 political context of the epidemic in South Africa, where despite high HIV prevalence, few people are open about their status, the division between owning and buying HIV knowledge and experience can seem more salient than nice distinctions between commercial and academic appropriations. I leave the meeting expecting there to be little followup. However, the next day one woman calls and invites me to come to her support group to talk about the research. She thinks the fee is acceptable, and she and her friends have things that they want to say.

A few days later I meet with members of another HIV-focused CBO, some of whom have already volunteered to be interviewed. The offices are busy with volunteers and paid workers advising people who walk in with questions or problems, holding meetings, telephoning and helping visitors like myself. As at the other organisation, all the volunteers and paid workers are black. The coordinator tells me that so far, despite invitations, white South Africans have been slow to get involved. These interviewees ask me to use their real names when I write up the research; they want to be open about their status. I say that one of the ethical conditions of the research is anonymisation. Since it is important for some participants, we need to provide it for all. In addition, circumstances may change, and what a participant says openly now may have a different significance for them in future. Such research criteria mean little in the present political context of this CBO, which foregrounds 'owning' HIV in the sense of being open about one's HIV status. Some interviewees who are volunteers with the organisation, but otherwise unemployed, are doubtful about taking the fee, although they could certainly do with the money. They decide in the end to donate it back to the organisation. One interviewee, however, tells me that it will give him value in his family – where his HIV means he is now treated as a nobody – to come home with money for talking about HIV.

Speaking out about HIV is an important though problematic aspect of the South African epidemic. It can be difficult, dangerous and ineffective; but for many people, it seems vital – physically, psychologically and socially. It may even, as we saw in the last chapter, be the grounds for people's ethical and spiritual standing as HIV subjects. This chapter looks in more detail at the political implications of 'owning' the virus: at how people move in their representations of HIV from being accepting, open and ethical subjects, to being active, political subjects. As in the examples above, these moves may include 'owning' HIV as a commodity, and 'owning' it as a form of citizenly identification. Whichever route you take, making your relationship to HIV, as someone either infected or affected, a foundation of your speech as a political subject is a necessary basis for broader political talk about the epidemic. Without speaking subjects, HIV cannot be spoken of politically; it does not exist. Such silence is a familiar position in the history of many HIV epidemics. But it is not just a matter of declaring your HIV positive or HIV-affected status. An analysis of the power relations of HIV 'ownership' is also important in people's understanding of the condition. It is the *kind* of HIV citizenship that is declared and 'owned', and the relations it posits with other citizens, that determines the political shape of the epidemic.

'A normal person just like anybody'

So far this book has examined how people with HIV represent their lives as social and ethical subjects. Yet 'representation' has political meanings, too. The politics of people's personal narrative representations appear in what precisely is said, by whom, and to whom. In 'speaking out' as HIV subjects in the research, for instance, the interviewees were talking to us as researchers, but also to the wider possible audiences for the research – other people living with HIV, NGOs and CBOs, policy-makers and the future readers of an archive. Often, embedded in their stories were accounts of how they had described themselves to others – sisters, partners, friends.

I want to start by concentrating on how interviewees told stories of themselves as 'a normal person just like anybody', to use David's words. These stories, positioning them in relation to other citizens, articulated forms of HIV citizenship and ownership that constituted the basis for their other, more explicitly political speech. In these stories, our interviewees demonstrated the conditions of subjecthood that are linked to claims to HIV ownership.[1]

The foundation for being a citizen 'just like anybody' is that you are the same person as you were before you knew your HIV status. David, telling the 'very short' story of his life with HIV since his recent diagnosis, for instance, specified this identity early in the interview:

> **David**: I must tell you that I was waiting for bad results because I've known myself, I've been, I haven't been safe. I mean I haven't been playing safe over the years, so I was really expecting bad news, so I was waiting for those bad news. And the results came and I was tested HIV positive. Okay, there's that little bit of a shock. Yes, there is, but it didn't change me. I, I used to have dreams and I still have. Being HIV positive, I mean didn't change all those dreams. I'm still me and I'll always be me.

This declaration of identity, 'I'm still me', did not involve an evasion of the impact of HIV or the changes it could make. 'I've known myself . . . I haven't been safe,' David said. David was also one of the interviewees who talked most about what would happen to his health in future, and about how other, iller people managed their lives. Nor was he declaring himself the same as all other citizens. Rather, his declarations worked to position David as not equal but democratically *equivalent* to other citizens. Such equivalence was asserted by many other interviewees, for instance, Busisiwe, whose reported description to her friends of any woman living with HIV as 'a person amongst others', begins this book. Chantal Mouffe (1993: 84) argues that such equivalence allows grounds for commonality and resistance to be built and political associations to be made (Walzer, 1983) while also acknow-ledging important conditions of difference – in this case, in health status. The CBO member who suggested a R350 interview fee was certainly arguing for equivalence, not identity between people who were openly HIV positive citizens and others – indeed, they precisely costed the difference. That costing also suggested that the difference between HIV positive people and other equally poor, and perhaps equally ill, citizens was a stigmatisation that was expensive to transcend. Certainly stigmatisation was, and continues to be, a reality for many people living with HIV in South Africa.

The second CBO, however, mapped differences between HIV positive and other citizens more widely, starting from health, and taking in not just stigmatisation, but also people's resistance to it through 'speaking out'. It set up a field of citizenly equivalence that allowed collective action, not just individualised reaction. Many of our interviewees were engaged in a similar political project of personal 'speaking out'.

Later in the interview, David explicitly presented himself in terms of a common humanity. This commonality seemed to relate to the concept of *ubuntu* sometimes cited by interviewees. But David was also using a 'rights' concept that is current internationally, in debates about 'human rights'. Mandela, too, invoked rights in his 2000 speech at the World AIDS Con-ference. Rights are now part of UNAIDS discourse (Piot, 2001), and are also an important focus of post-apartheid South African political discourse (Phillips, 2003). A claim can be made, for instance, across health statuses on the basis of the rights laid out in the Constitution. Generally, the interviewees did not treat rights abstractly but rather mentioned them in relation to specific objects such as medical treatment, housing and education – something that characterises 'rights' arguments in many developing-world social movements.[2]

Rights arguments therefore worked not just as descriptions and claims of identity – in this case, the identity of a citizen with an illness – but as identity 'ownership', as claims on certain objects to which that identity entitles you. The CBO member who asked for a R350 fee for every HIV positive person who did an interview, was making such a claim. But most interviewees' rights claims were broader, and not simply economic in nature. Instead, interviewees claimed, as HIV positive people, rights equivalent to those of other citizens, in the realms of, for instance, healthcare, employment and being treated 'like a person'.

Interviewees also pointed out their equivalence to non-HIV positive citizens outside a 'rights' framework, within an analysis of the conditions of their lives. Again, this frequently involved plans for education and employment, particularly among male interviewees who reported higher levels of education, like Michael:

> **Michael**: I think HIV didn't turn my, my goals /mhm/ or my expectation you know yah, I didn't told myself 'as I'm HIV positive I can't do this and this'. But ah, yah, in my life, I, I I told myself that if I can go I mean for my studies to become just engineering you know all those thing, but because of the money I don't have money, yah but the thing is that HIV didn't turn my goals and my expectations of life. I do normal things that I should be doing if I was positive, if I was negative you know.

Many interviewees made more wide-ranging analyses of their conditions of equivalence to non-HIV positive citizens, though these analyses were still pragmatically rooted in everyday concerns. Nosisi, for instance, who had another chronic illness as well as HIV, repeatedly argued that 'a person with HIV does not die quickly. S/he does not die of HIV either, rather of other diseases'. She enumerated the other life-threatening aspects of a poor environment – lack of food, flooding in your house, no heating, no clothes: 'I would say these are the kinds of things that kill a person.' In making this analysis, Nosisi was, again, not claiming that HIV makes no difference. She interweaved the analysis with accounts of her own involvement in HIV organisations and the need for specific provision for HIV positive people. She was, however, pointing to the often primary conditions of similarity between people of different HIV statuses when they are living in resource-constrained circumstances. In this context, spoken-out assertions of equivalence become the starting point for political demands, not for individual rights, but for larger programmes promoting social justice. In Nosisi's case, these demands related primarily to training and employment; she made them particularly, but not only, for those directly affected by the epidemic.

Interviewees' assertions of the citizenly equivalence of an HIV positive person to people of other statuses were often made in opposition to the abjection of HIV, which was represented through the words and reactions of others. When, for instance, Busisiwe declared that she and any other HIV positive woman should be viewed as 'a person amongst others', this claim followed her resistance of her friends' possible rejection of such women: 'People, HIV is not something that should make you dislike me . . . so, do not treat your sister as if she is no longer a person.' In the rest of the interview, Busisiwe recounted many instances of being treated as not 'a person' by her mother, who even now made her feel 'not at home'. Zoleka similarly described her planned disclosure to her family of her HIV positive status, 'I'm like this and like that', against the possibility of being 'looked down on' as an abject, physically repulsive other:

> **Zoleka**: Like now, I'm going home {to the countryside}. I haven't told anybody at home about my HIV status. I'm not keen to tell them over the phone. I want to tell my sisters and brothers. Sit down with them and explain to them that I'm like this and like that. 'Don't turn your backs on me, such that you would even hate the glass from which I drink water.'

Being 'a person amongst others' was, then, an equivalent identity re-counted – and in the process owned, though not always completely – in the face of abjection. This articulation of personhood was more foundational than David's description of being the same person as before, and having rights like other people, or Nosisi's account of the common material conditions of personhood. It claimed the very condition of being a person, 'a human being just like them' as David put it, for people with HIV.

Abjection and stigma are, as we saw in earlier chapters, at least partly socially produced phenomena. For our interviewees, they could be combatted within accounts of HIV personhood, through the presentation of a healthy, right-living, ethical self. For many interviewees like Zoleka, the point of disclosing your status 'in person' to your family was, indeed, to demonstrate that you were still a person, with good health and a positive state of mind, as well as being HIV positive. Others wanted to declare themselves HIV positive only when their babies had tested negative, or when they themselves had accessed successful treatment. They could become openly HIV positive citizens, therefore, only in the context of appropriate treatment availability. For many who do not get tested for HIV, it is undoubtedly the case that even personal knowledge of oneself as an HIV positive person is unthinkable outside the context of the treatment possibilities that could sustain such a person.

Other research participants, like Pam, narrated their HIV personhood not against the present possibilities, but against a future of universal HIV. Here, Pam opposes the imagined abjection of her expulsion from her family, by picturing to them the increasingly HIV-affected futures of all families:

> **Pam**: I've told {my family}, my parents accepted it /mhm/ my brothers, my sisters accepted it, there, there's there was not change, but it was hard /mhm . . . and they do understand that in 2004 each and every family will have a person who's suffering from this virus /mhm/ and it's a disaster and there is no cure /mhm/ so they can't just chuck me out.

Pam describes, realistically, a 'disaster' of incurable and untreated illness by 2004. Such teleological narratives were not apocalyptic. Rather, they formed grounds of shared personhood and citizenship on which action about the epidemic could be taken, across HIV statuses. Interviews with the gate-keepers for this research project, who were HIV negative or of unknown HIV status, produced some similar formulations of equivalent citizenship, which refused ideologically to distinguish between the HIV positive and people who are HIV affected but negative or of unknown status, while emphasising the practical significance of these distinctions. For one non-HIV positive gatekeeper, this identification even led to weakened links with non-HIV-involved friends. He was part of an HIV citizenship that was clearly defined by political interest, not HIV status:

> **Themba:** It's good to see {friends} from time to time but the problem is, they take things light. They have not been there with me and seen people really dying of HIV and AIDS /mhm/ and it has frustrated me because it's it is as if it's too far from them and, and, and some of their discussions are not, are not, are superficial on issues that are confronting the country.

Such failures of HIV citizenship could, in interviewees' accounts, be found, to a degree, among HIV positive people themselves: in the destructive silence and isolation of the diagnosed people that Benjamin described; among Busisiwe's friends and ex-boyfriend, seeing partners and children dying, ill themselves, yet refusing even to test; and sometimes among people who had 'accepted' their own status like Michael's girlfriend, but who could not bear a broader identity as an HIV positive person, like that brought on her by his advocacy work.

At the same time, interviewees acknowledged the frequent closeness of relations between HIV positive people, particularly shortly after diagnosis – relationships that emerged clearly in earlier chapters' descriptions of the reflective intimacy of support groups. Some of our interviewees themselves noted that they had at first assumed that such relationships would be the only ones available to them as HIV subjects, since HIV negative people would reject them. Yoliswa, for example, described herself in this position after diagnosis:

> **Yoliswa**: During the first months of finding out, the HIV people were the only people that I thought were very close to me ... I tried to distance the HIV negative people because I thought they were terrible to us.

Even later, there were elements of HIV life that some interviewees thought could only be shared with other HIV positive people. Michael, for instance, had had HIV negative girlfriends, but he thought they were 'doing a favour' to him. He wanted a relationship with a woman who was positive and had a thought-out, open approach to her status:

Michael: I'm looking for someone who's HIV positive and the girlfriend should be should be proud of herself, she should be open about her status, and she should be, she should be her own be yourself and all those things, I want a girlfriend who's open about status and she should be very strong.

The closed 'citizenships' of exclusively HIV positive subjects that interviewees articulated were momentary, reactive and partial. However, they need to be noted against any assumption that the equivalence of HIV and other subjectivities can be reduced to an equation of identity between them.

Politically speaking

When people constituted themselves as citizens in an HIV polity in the ways I've described, they claimed political ownership of the condition. They were pragmatic about this; few were openly HIV positive in all situations, they were not *only* HIV subjects, and they did not assume identity between everyone with HIV. Rather, HIV citizenship was an equivalent position, and they were ready to negotiate this position in relation to citizens with other claims. How did such HIV citizens explicitly address politics? In Chapter 3 I looked at how people described political structures supporting their lives with HIV, and in Chapter 4, at how such structures operated at times as 'interpretive communities' within which people took on personal ownership of their HIV positive lives. In the South African context, where, more explicitly than in many other countries, HIV is a political as well as a health issue, the relation of HIV lives to politics needs a more direct address. First, though, it is important to sketch something of the general political framing of the epidemic.

The South African epidemic's political saturation can be seen at every level, from international reports and continuing parliamentary controversy, down to everyday talk about the condition. In public life, 'rights' talk – drawing on international law, the constitution and local formulations of entitlements, like that constructed by David – coexist with more nation-specific traditions of rhetoric drawn from the anti-apartheid struggle and the Truth and Reconciliation Commission. The church and contemporary political parties and organisations contribute to this political language. The managerial political languages of international health and development organisations, the personalised, consumption-orientated political languages of transnational popular culture, and discourses of African and broader developing-world politics and activism also feed into the political language of HIV.

While it is often expected that the struggle against apartheid provides the foundational legacy for current activism, including HIV activism, there is no simple correspondence between such traditions and effective HIV politics. Some individuals, communities and groups active in the anti-apartheid struggle have translated their activism into the HIV field; others have dissociated this history from HIV activism. The divergences between activists formed in different periods of the anti-apartheid struggle those who were in jail and those who were not, those who stayed in South Africa and those who left, place of exile (different countries within Africa, the Soviet bloc, Europe, the US), those who came into government and those who did not, between women and men, and between activists from different provinces and of different ethnicities, all play into different political takes on the HIV epidemic. So do historic divisions between organisations within the anti-apartheid movement, and between organisations in and outside the movement, for instance between the ANC and the Inkatha Freedom Party and the Democratic Alliance, whose main bases of support are respectively in KwaZulu-Natal and the Western Cape.[3]

Competing claims for the anti-apartheid legacy occur within the HIV field. The Treatment Action Campaign, TAC, the most well-known South African HIV activist organisation, has tried to avoid generalised political conflict with the government. Many of its members are indeed also members of the governing ANC. However, when in 2001 TAC used a photograph of Nkosi Johnson alongside an image of Hector Pieterson, the 13-year-old killed in the Soweto uprisings, in a campaign for MTCT treatment, it drew a somewhat incendiary parallel between the apartheid regime's violent suppression of these uprisings and the contemporary failure to provide ARV treatment for pregnant women – treatment which was then being opposed by the ANC, the very party that had fought apartheid. Later, TAC described the health and trade and industry ministers as 'murderers'. This campaign, however, also drew, both visually and textually, on 'wanted' posters from ACT UP's New York late-1980s 'Reagan kills me', Cardinal O'Connor 'Public Health Menace' and Wellcome 'AIDS Profiteer' campaigns (Crimp and Ralston, 1990). This link is just one of the most obvious transnational representational connection between South African and other epidemics' HIV activism. TAC's concurrent civil disobedience campaigns involving picketing and street demonstrations also recalled ACT UP actions, but in addition, a long tradition of anti-apartheid civil disobedience including the Defiance Campaign against the Pass Laws in the 1950s. TAC's campaign against pharmaceutical companies' monopoly, the Christopher Moraka Defiance Campaign, deliberately referred to that precedent. All this meant that TAC's activism could be understood by national and international audiences in ways that went beyond simple anti-government responses, linking it historically and sociopolitically to other forms of resistance. At the same time, it organised transnationally, founding a set of support organisations in developed countries, and establishing links with other developing countries that were already mobilizing for treatment, in and beyond Africa (Iliffe, 2006: 155).[4]

At the province level, there are salient differences in HIV politics. HIV policies in the Western Cape, where we did our research, are perhaps most divergent from the national picture and have become influential templates for the rest of the country and internationally. This province has been helped in developing its effective policies by having relatively few HIV cases among inhabitants defined as coloured and white, although rates among black Africans in the province are similar to those elsewhere in the country. The Western Cape is, in addition, relatively wealthy, with well-developed periurban health and social services. Its health HIV policy may also have been politically enabled because it is historically less allied to the ANC, and thus was less institutionally and personally tied to government HIV policies. All this has allowed the development and implementation of well-planned and community-responsive HIV healthcare – and gender – policies, different to that seen nationally (Abdullah *et al.*, 2006; Gouws, 2006). The Democratic Alliance, still the main national opposition party, was indeed in government in the Western Cape when my research started.

Many organisations and communities not connected to the freedom struggle, or formed after it, have been at the forefront of HIV activism. At least 34 per cent of the population was born after 1992, so the percentage of people for whom apartheid is a clear memory is rapidly diminishing (Statistics South Africa, 2001). Many now live, as was the case for most of our interviewees, in informal settlements of recent origin with a relatively new history of community organisation. In some provinces, particularly Guateng, 'pro-poor' campaigns opposed to the government, and drawing on political and community organisations, many with quite recent histories, are strongly linked to HIV activism.

Nevertheless, the country's powerful tradition of anti-apartheid education, organisation and action does seem to shape HIV politics, locally and nationally, beyond the personal histories of some of the activists involved. While Archbishop Tutu and others have called for a strengthening of this connection, it may be that it is already powerful, albeit implicitly. Pragmatic forms of thinking and action, like those developing around HIV, draw, as West (1989) points out, not only on the immediacies and intricacies of contemporary situations, but also on 'traditions' of resistance and change.

What of the new political field of 'speaking out' about HIV – where did this come from? 'Speaking out' is a nation-building genre in South Africa, with a long political history, as indeed it is in other countries that engaged in twentieth-century struggles against colonialism. Most recently, the genre appeared in the country's saturation with stories from the Truth and Reconciliation Commission (Edelstein, 2002; Gobodo-Madikizela, 2003; Krog, 2000; Truth and Reconciliation Commission and Tutu, 1999). The genre is also exhibited through the increasing volume and multiplicity of voices heard in the country since the rout of the apartheid government, and foreshadowed in the long preceding struggle for an effective voice. Nkosi Johnson, when he told his story to the 2000 International AIDS Conference, spoke as a direct descendant both of the recent TRC storytelling, and of that much longer struggle to have your voice heard. Interviewees, who spoke to us in the period just before and after Johnson's death, sometimes used his public storytelling as an explicit model for their own speech. It could be argued that they too were speaking in the cultural context of the recent TRC hearings, and, for some of them, of the personal voices in the anti-apartheid struggle.

Testimonies from the Truth and Reconciliation Commission were ubiquitous in South African media in the mid-1990s. In May 2006, invoking this precedent, and bemoaning South Africa's failure fully to address the HIV epidemic as it had the legacy of apartheid, the *Lancet* called in a high profile editorial for a 'TRC' for the epidemic. However, during the TRC's later stages, when dealing with reparation, the government posed the TRC *against* pressing issues of the 'present' such as HIV, which it viewed as likely to overwhelm the TRC (Reparation and Rehabiliation Committee, 2003). South Africans' sense of the value and justice of the TRC is ambiguous (Centre for the Study of Violence and Reconciliation and Khulamani Support Group, n.d). There is perhaps a more clearly effective history of autobiographical and biographical testimony during apartheid itself, in the works of, for instance, Ezekial Mphaphlele (1959), Desmond Tutu (2006 [1989]), Steve Biko (1996), Bessie Head (1968), Ellen Kuzwayo (2004 [1985]), Winnie Madikizela-Mandela (Mandela. W., 1985), and Nelson Mandela (1995). Some of this writing is coloured by the religious structures of conversion and witnessing discussed in the previous chapter. Some is framed in terms of legal rights, within which it becomes testimony explicitly in the interests of justice – for instance, testimony on removals, detentions and killings, like the documentation of the imprisonment and killing of Steve Biko (for instance, Bernstein, 1978).[5] Some is fictional and poetic, transmuting personal experiences into dramatic and ethical narratives (Ndebele, 1994).

A less frequently invoked but also clear precedent for the politics of openness is lesbian and gay activism, whose effects on not just the Treatment Action Campaign, through key members involved in sexual identity politics, but also on other HIV organisations in the country, have been considerable (Heywood, 2005; Mbali, 2005). 'Coming out' is not the model for HIV speech it has very often been in developed-world countries. There, HIV positive heterosexual women and men in the early years of epidemics frequently 'learned' openness and self-acceptance within support groups established by gay men, many of whom had addressed similar issues about sexual identities in the 1960s and 1970s (Squire, 1999). In South Africa, the politics of HIV disclosure drew less directly on the politics of 'coming out'. However, the politics of ACT UP on which TAC and, less directly other South African HIV organizations, draw was itself derived from post-Stonewall lesbian and gay activism in the US. Moreover, our interviewees were aware of the excluded early voices of the pandemic in South Africa and elsewhere, of people they had characterised early in the epidemic as not 'like' them, sexually and often also racially and nationally. Interviewees' contemporary insistence on human commonality seemed indeed at times an implicit revision of these exclusions. Interviewees usually made such revisions indirectly, in brief asides about the similarities they had realised in the face of HIV, between 'different' people the world over. Sometimes, they asserted a quasi-familial equivalence between themselves and HIV campaigners who were demographically unlike them, including in some instances in their sexualities – for instance, in several cases referring to local gay HIV gay campaigners as their 'brother' or 'father'. Family metaphors and similes are common in South Africans' speech; they are powerful ways of establishing commonalities across sexual identities.[6] Some interviewees also spoke directly of their enlightening experiences in groups earlier in the epidemic that included white and black gay men as well as heterosexual black Africans, of developing HIV understanding and campaigns across sexualities and racialised categories.

The powerful history of struggle autobiographies, the public ubiquity of TRC testimony and the discourse of 'coming out' may, then, have had effects in constructing 'speaking out' as a form of political action for our inter-viewees. Nevertheless, the precedents for speaking out that they noted were much more specific to HIV: Nkosi Johnson's speech, Mandela's declara-tions, other public figures' disclosures of their status, soap fiction and talk show discussions.

Whatever its antecedents, 'speaking out' has become a new form of political activism, the most distinct within the HIV field and the latest move in South Africa's revolutionary political trajectory. This politicised mode of talking about HIV, emblematised in support groups, has important effects of its own, in creating social and sometimes virtual communities of HIV support that can be overtly political. The groups bring together people of different genders; classes (although in this research, few were middle class); ages, from teenage years into the forties; of varying linguistic, regional, cultural and political backgrounds (among these interviewees, people recently arrived in Cape Town from the Eastern Cape, people who had lived in the Western Cape for many years, and a few Zulu-speaking people from KwaZulu-Natal). The groups negotiate HIV citizenship across these differences, without erasing them. Interviewees' comments on people's backgrounds and econo-mic statuses in particular clarified their awareness of these differences within the HIV citizenship that they were developing. In addition, for women, the groups seemed to articulate a gender politics that helped them deal with stigmatising family members and bad relationships, and these politics were practised in the interviews. A woman who spoke of leaving the man who beat her was met with approving murmurs and nods by the support group acquaintances interviewed with her. Andiswa, the woman who lived with her sister to avoid her boyfriend but was still dependent on his money, and who had not told any family members her status, was tactfully advised by her friend Zukiswa to begin disclosing to her family, start saving, and become independent:

Zukiswa: The person with the virus, can call that person {family member} to come to the clinic. Maybe three or rather four of them, with two nurses . . . I mean in her position, I am thinking for her,

> because I can't lie, if parents know, that makes me feel alright and
> safe . . . During my pregnancy I used to stay with my sister up there.
> While I lived there my boyfriend used to give me money, so I saved
> the money and deposited it on a bangalo {wooden shack} until I
> finished. I put it there, and I live by myself now.

The most powerful effects of speaking out happen when, as Plummer
(1995) describes, interpretive communities become communities of social
action. A number of more politically active and longer-diagnosed interviewees described the limits on the HIV citizenship reached in groups.
Phumla, for instance, wanted to leave her group that just 'sat' and 'stand up
and be part of the people who are fighting for people's rights'. Michael found
the groups too negative, not forward-looking enough. Similarly, 'speaking
out' to narrow audiences of families and friends could be constraining
when they refused, or were too overwhelmed, to hear you. Benjamin and
Busisiswe, after talking to daughters and mothers, respectively, who turned
a deaf ear, were seeking more political engagement as speaking HIV citizens.

At the same time, even simply 'speaking out' about HIV is still not always
possible. The effects of all the local and national HIV organisations and
services working to enable HIV talk and action must be set against the
still-powerful constraints on people's hearing and telling of tales of personal and political resistance to HIV. These constraints are partly those
encountered throughout the pandemic, of medical intractability, generalized
stigma, gendered discrimination, and competing priorities in resource-
restricted situations. Apartheid also contributed to the economic, educational and political context of the South African epidemic. Subsequently,
international commercial profiteering, and the ineffectualness and negligence
of the development and AIDS industries have enhanced the difficulties, as has
the country's own history of political inaction and policy inertia. Discussing
continuing high rates of new infections, Zackie Achmat, quoted at the
beginning of this chapter, spreads blame appropriately widely over 'governments, international agencies, business, the scientific community, faith-based
organizations, civil society bodies, communities and individuals' (2006).

How did our research participants talk about such politics? Eight
interviewees talked explicitly about political campaigns about HIV, including advocacy or activism to change the policies of drug companies and
government. Often these openly political references were quite brief,
occurring as part of more general stories about interviewees' modes of living
with the virus. Benjamin, for example, who had been diagnosed for almost
ten years, described his life as a very politically active one, involving
considerable amounts of time spent in community education and advocacy.
He explained that 'I manage to, to, to help the President to fight Glaxo and
Pfizer to distribute these tablets'. The other seven interviewees who talked
directly about politics, articulated far-reaching understandings of the HIV
politics of the government, the WHO, international pharmaceutical com-

panies and generic drug companies operating elsewhere in the developing world. Like Benjamin, they explicated these politics pragmatically, in conjunction with accounts of local demonstrations, the particular treatment failures of neighbourhood clinics, and the preventable deaths of friends and family.

Four of the group who spoke explicitly about politics, all older inter-viewees, related HIV politics to other community or political activism by referring to past activism or to their contemporary work in other community groups. Mary, for instance, addressed the tape recorder at several points in the interview to deliver judgements about the government and to make a final pronouncement in a style loaned from a long history of activism:

> **Mary**: All I want to say is: forward with {organisation name}! It's {organisation name} that I value highly, rather than this government of ours which is asleep.

Such accounts, though conventionally 'political' in their vocabulary and their thematic emphases on struggle and change, were again grounded in everyday difficulties and possibilities, and able to address the ambiguities these produced. Benjamin's accounts of his very partial successes in edu-cating both young people and men his own age about HIV were exemplary. In the middle of a long description of the difficulties, he described these audiences to his 'speaking out' about HIV as 'water in an open hand'.

Typically of younger interviewees who addressed politics directly, Yoliswa, who had discovered her HIV status in the aftermath of her baby's diagnosis, illness and death in 1999, described speaking to the media and the public on HIV issues, but presented these actions in personalised ways, using little obviously political language. Yoliswa was, in fact, an early and effec-tive public representative of the case for antiretroviral treatment for pregnant women, but her interview descriptions were very largely about the personal impact of this activism. 'I so wish there can be MTCT for other mothers' was as close as she came to a direct political statement about the issue. Recounting her engagement with an advocacy organisation, she described how this involvement gave her back to herself as – like David – the 'same' person she had previously been:

> **Yoliswa**: I think meeting {HIV organisation} had a very very big impact on my life ... I stopped having the negative thoughts and, just started to be the old Yoliswa I used to be before I knew about my HIV status.

She also gave an extended, and again personally focused, account of perceived government neglect of the epidemic, naming individuals, specu-lating about their feelings and relating them to how people with HIV themselves feel:

Yoliswa: Manto Tshabalala {Minister of Health} once said that this HIV shouldn't be a priority, there are other priorities as well.The people living with HIV think that the HIV is a priority because people are dying in big numbers and that is affecting the economy of the country but they {government} don't say it as something that could be considered first. So, this government of ours doesn't care if we die or not because, I remember one day Nkosi {Johnson} invited this President of ours but he never showed up but instead he sent his wife. She didn't even hug the boy just to show that as government they care. She just went there and nothing else so, they just don't care. I don't know, maybe because they know they are not positive and they won't be positive, I don't know. They just don't feel this as and I think maybe if it was still Madiba {Mandela} in the throne, maybe things will be better. Yah I think so, at least that man has feelings for other people, and maybe he would have done something.

Many interviewees expressed a similarly negative take on political institutions in their comments about the social exclusion of people with HIV. They said that the world had forgotten them, drug companies and the international community did not mind if they died, the HIV negative just wanted them to go away, and the government didn't care, either *that* they existed – since HIV was conceptualised only as an adjunct of poverty – or *how* they existed. This discourse of anti-politics was dissipated by material provision, as the much more favourable descriptions of government policy from women on MTCT programmes demonstrate. However, it may be that prolonged political disappointment about HIV will create a sustained disengagement that adds to that already produced by other perceived political failures and betrayals.

Perhaps more significant than this negatively formulated politics, though, was that, as with Yoliswa, many interviewees' political narratives were formulated around their own experiences and feelings, a form of 'political' speech not immediately associated with South Africa. When such personalised or emotivist (MacIntyre, 1984) speech is described in the developed world, it is often said to be non-political, an abdication of politics for selfhood. At the same time, such language is becoming a recognized form of political expression within 'post-political' western democracies (Goodwin *et al.*, 2001). Within developed-world HIV politics, personal testimony has also long operated both as activism and as memory (Watney, 2000). The ANC's partial reinvention as a 'modern', technocratic party, against its previous popular identification with the nation (Gumede, 2005), may have contributed to the personalisation of political language, while at the same time creating a space within everyday culture, once occupied by politics, now filled with more individualised concerns.

In our research, 'speaking out' about your HIV status, despite the problems and limitations sometimes associated with it in support groups and families, could indeed be a powerful political strategy, claiming as it did a personhood held in common across HIV statuses. The equivalent HIV 'self' that our interviewees articulated, with common humanity, equal rights and full political status, but specific HIV-related requirements, was never simply a psychological one. And it was always in negotiation with the silent, abjected non-self or non-person of people's fears, for its citizenly existence. Acceptance of and openness about this HIV self worked to affirm the existence of HIV, against the 'lightness,' the non-existence or inconsequentiality, which was until around 2000 ascribed to it. Just as HIV secrecy and denial were historically linked, both politically and personally, so, in this research, were 'speaking out' and the possibility of political action around HIV. Linda gave a clear account of these connections when, having listened to an acquaintance, Phumla, describe how she wanted to move out from her support group to help similar young mothers, she formulated her own project in response:

> **Linda**: I find it important that as the other lady has mentioned it that we should go places to help people. I think it is important to give personal examples when you talk to people, so that the weak can become stronger and learn from you that you are also strong. When you encourage people you must encourage them with what they see in you ... It is also important if the government could provide accommodation for HIV positive people that have been chased out of their homes because they disclosed their status to their families. If we could have a place to accommodate them and make them feel welcomed, I think that is very important.

Linda's story of how her future HIV engagement should go is constructed in dialogue with Phumla's more concrete recommendations, which included suggestions for remunerating community workers. Linda too proposes practical 'help', even a government structure of collective housing, and a kind of witnessing that has some religious antecedents. But her account rests on personal 'speaking out' and its strengthening effects, and making HIV positive people feel 'welcomed', against their self-stigmatisation, familial exile and abjectification.

'Speaking out' about HIV, if only in some cases to oneself and, in our study, to the researchers and the tape recorder, thus seemed to operate as a significant political affirmation of a citizenly identity from which people perceived themselves as in danger of exclusion. This exclusion worked, first through general, although culturally variable, patterns of stigma and silencing around HIV, and second, through more specific South African political representations of HIV as 'other' (Joffe, 1997), and as a condition of poverty, that also turned people with HIV into non-citizens. Interviewees' own frequent representations of HIV positive people's political exclusion bore witness to this pattern, as did many participants' surprise that people from places 'outside' their neighbourhoods had come to listen to them.

In participants' stories of themselves as political subjects and of political action, then, a direct claim to membership in the local, national and international political body was made. The stories turned the interviewees from the social and ethical subjects of the previous chapter, accepting, open and positive about their HIV status, into speaking, political subjects, engaged in pragmatic negotiation between the everyday contingencies of their lives and principles of equity and justice, and, often, pursuing these negotiations through personal disclosure narratives. Though these stories were individually formulated, they were 'testimonial' stories, both for the speakers and their audience as Plummer (2001) has described this category. Bernstein described her account of the life and death of Steven Biko as a 'magnifying glass', through which 'a whole spectrum of South African reality is exposed' (1978: 7). Many South African autobiographies work similarly. As exemplary accounts of national or more locally political lives, they transmit past realities to their readers, and suggest future possibilities to them (Koyana, 2001).[7] Our interviewees, too, were describing conditions shared by many, in circumstances where only a few could speak. Often, interviewees individually and in groups, told stories in a common voice, as narratives of a collective, or a 'community of selves' (Ogbonnaya, 1994; Plummer, 2001: 31). Such stories described shared HIV realities that should not be forgotten, and that could help others who heard them to address their own futures.

These stories of political but highly personalised HIV subjects thus used a new, situation-specific political language for talking about HIV in South Africa. It seems a particularly useful language for younger people who are proxy speakers of South Africa's older political language, and for whom older political languages do not seem compelling. This newer language may allow a form of subjectively-focused, 'conscientising' dialogue (Holdstock, 2000:138) already politically recognised as important in South African youth media, for instance, through the series *Yizo Yizo* (Barnett, 1994). Perhaps this language is also helpful for women, whose relation to older political languages has often been ambiguous.[8] Perhaps, too, such language provides new possibilities of transnational understandings. Grounded here in highly particular politics, its emotionalised character is nevertheless understood and used in many global contexts, its commonality driven by increasing access to globalised media. Researchers generally explore the transnational aspects of popular organisations through documented policy links between relatively formal and politically orientated organisations such as TAC, rather than through language. Even at this activist level, though, researchers increasingly recognise the emotionality of such discourse and action (Goodwin *et al.*, 2001). TAC's own use of contextualised personal stories has expanded recently, in particular to support womens's rights work. The WHO's adoption in its recent HIV initiatives of similarly contextualized personal testimony in their 'Voices of Hope' photostories,[9] attests to the mainstream policy recognition of the significance of such narratives.

People's narratives of HIV were, in addition to being personal stories of personal circumstances, overdetermined affirmations of political existence, asserted against both the general stigmatisation and silencing of HIV, and the more particular history of HIV's political erasure in South Africa. At the same time, the stories usefully indicate difficult aspects of HIV that cannot be dealt with in interpretive 'communities'. These difficulties include the abjection of HIV that cannot completely be come to terms with. They also include what I have called the 'equivalent' aspects of HIV citizenship, that is, the disjunctions that break up equations between the HIV positive and the HIV negative, the HIV infected and affected and those not affected, and that operate between HIV positive people themselves. The stories thus exemplify a more general tension between citizenly equivalence and its limits within democratic political structures (MacIntyre, 1984). That tension has particular relevance for people with HIV, who, even in situations of high prevalence are in danger of internal exclusion within democratic structures. In these interviews, people built pragmatic political associations with 'equivalent' others by speaking from a foundation of citizenly HIV equivalence, where people with HIV were 'just like anybody'. As one gatekeeper, not known to be HIV positive but assuming this identification, put it:

> **Zanele**: Even now I take myself as an HIV person because I don't know my status /mhm/ that is why I told myself that maybe I've got this HIV. So I, I'm on the side of HIV people. I don't say I'm not or I will not, I take myself as an HIV person.

HIV was, moreover, about to become everyone's issue, one from which you cannot secrete yourself or your family, or escape by youth or age:

> **Benjamin**: Next day it gonna be there in your family /mhm/ Because you're not gonna lock the gates and go to work /mhm/ and come and open the gates. /mhm/ One mistake there'll be HIV it's just like a death /mhm/ as we say most death is visiting families to families. So it's just like the case of HIV /mhm/ Don't put it as the issue of the teenagers. It starts from zero to sixty to beyond you see.

HIV is thus now – like death – a fact of life. But Benjamin accurately presents the risks of other health issues that visit 'families to families' as also high. The equivalence of everyone in the face of HIV is, he suggests, as with these other life-threatening phenomena, the condition of future social existence.

Conclusion

HIV futures

One and a half million people are on antiretroviral therapy in the developing world. And hopefully there will be far more. Twenty, 30 or 40 years from now, we still want them to be alive. Who's going to pay for that? Let's start thinking in terms of decades and generations.

Peter Piot, Executive Director, UNAIDS,
2006 World AIDS Conference, Toronto, *Guardian*, 14 August 2006

Many of us working to alleviate the impact of AIDS are alarmed that, despite our best efforts, we have not yet turned the tide of AIDS. To do this we must all make a serious commitment to promote long-term solutions not quick fixes. It could mean challenging some long-standing customs and traditions, reforming outdated legal systems. It means changing the way the world works and it won't be easy. However, if we value women, and if we are committed to stopping AIDS, it's not just the right thing to do – it's the smart thing to do.

Graça Machel and Kathleen Cravero, 2004

Yoliswa: I just want to go and live in a flat with my child and have a car that's all I want now. Having a car, whoo, if I can just get employed the first thing I will buy it's a car. I never wanted or in fact had a feeling of having a car before but now I want it.

Interviewer: So that you can go where, where would you go, why is it so important to you?

Yoliswa: Everywhere. Whenever I want to take my child to {the seaside}, I will just take my child in my car and go with him. I just want to give him the best while I'm still here because he's my only thing.

Consider the following problem, derived from a real-life situation in the South African epidemic's second decade.

A group of local women have been providing low-cost playgroup care for children in a resource-poor neighbourhood for some time. The group becomes aware of increasing numbers of parents dying from AIDS-related illnesses. They approach a local NGO working with HIV and AIDS for help. This NGO provides the organisation with a comprehensive plan for supporting AIDS-affected families, and helps the women form a trust. Then it finds foreign donors who want to help children affected by AIDS. The project gets funding for day care for HIV-infected and affected children, and for a pre-school, in line with the government's plans to develop early childhood education.

As the epidemic progresses, the original group of women decide that the neighbourhood is now as a whole 'HIV affected', and that it is stigmatising to identify certain children as HIV positive. In addition, in a situation where everyone is 'living with HIV' but where there is also severe unemployment, they argue that they must serve parents who have jobs but no childcare. Moreover, they must employ as many local people as possible as childcare workers, rather than giving their money to fewer, more qualified pre-school teachers. The programme will then support the neighbourhood's economic development, but will not deliver the 'pre-school education' its funders wanted, and its focus on all the children in the area means it will serve relatively few AIDS-affected children.

The trustees and funders object. They insist on giving priority to AIDS-affected families, and on employing some workers with qualifications in early childhood education. The women running the project and the employees demonstrate outside the facility, trying to reinstate their vision of how the project should run.

Although democratically organised, the group of women does not represent the whole community. It does not, in particular, represent all the AIDS-affected adults and children in the neighbourhood. Children who are HIV positive, or whose parents are ill with or have died from HIV, often have distinct social, emotional and educational requirements. AIDS-affected children and families are, in addition, the legal, named beneficiaries of the trust which now manages the project.

A local advocacy organisation for people living with HIV is invited to join the trust and to mediate with the disaffected playgroup project members. They compile a list of local HIV positive children and their needs. The women receive training around particular requirements of AIDS-affected and vunerable children. Parents of healthy children, aware that their children's presence in the pre-school is excluding children whose specific requirements they now recognise, find other local pre-schools. A compromise is reached. The group accepts AIDS-affected children into vacant places in the school and the programe continues with AIDS-affected families being prioritised.

The South African epidemic's early problems of silence, stigmatisation and lack of treatment continue today. Treatment rollout remains slow, particularly in rural areas. However, the dispute just described belongs to a new generation of problems concerning the pragmatic negotiation of HIV's equivalent citizenship in everyday contexts. HIV positive children are now receiving treatment, becoming healthier and living longer. HIV positive adults taking ARVs are living with and not dying from HIV; yet the drugs do not restore them to perfect health and economic productivity. They may lose their disability grant, but still find work difficult, if they are lucky enough to have some. Childcare may also be a strain. Sometimes, the drugs are difficult to take, have problematic side-effects or fail. This generation of problems will, as the UNAIDS Executive Director emphasises, last a long time. It arises from the fact that people living with HIV are equivalent, but not identical, to those who are not. They have specific requirements which even antiretroviral treatment does not remove.

In the example described above, providing resources for a particular group in a resource-poor situation had, as is common in such projects, skewing effects. In the developed world, too, providing grants, transport and food for HIV positive people who are resource-poor – for instance drug users, migrants and the urban unemployed – can generate conflicts. Other resource-poor people, not directly affected by HIV, see the provision as inequitable. They may grow irritated at hearing about HIV so much when they have so many other problems themselves. They may even claim that people who say they are HIV positive are lying to benefit from others' concern. Moreover, conflicts often occur when, as here, small, neighbourhood- or community-based HIV associations expand, acquiring paid workers, a governance structure, and external funding, all of which produce new stakeholders, each with a say in the organisation.

The real-life solution to the dispute above bridged divisions by acknowledging people's own realities, but also presenting them with the realities of HIV. The advocacy organisation managed, as our interviewees often reported doing themselves, to educate people not directly affected by HIV, about what its specific effects are. In response, the group of women who had initiated the project accepted some of the costs to their own autonomy and ways of working that came along with collaborating with larger NGOs and foreign funders, in the service of building the kind of neighbourhood project they did, indeed, want to be a part of. As Machel and Cravero suggest, established notions – in this case, about who the 'community' was and what its members' differing requirements were – had to change, to take into account the specificities of HIV positive lives. In addition, a neighbourhood association had to make compromise agreements with provincial and international organisations with differing structures and ideologies and greater power, in the interests of their shared commitment to helping HIV-affected families.

'Mainstreaming' HIV services into a menu of general concerns frequently arises as an alternative to HIV-oriented services like those described above. Mainstreaming carries its own difficulties of marginalising and short-changing people's HIV-related requirements (Elsey *et al.*, 2005). Nevertheless, the integration of HIV programmes into education (Matthews *et al.*, 2006), social services and primary health care, and the integration of HIV prevention and treatment programmes with each other (UNAIDS, 2006), are key features of current international and national HIV policies. Advocacy texts call for this integration. Mahlangu-Ngcobo's ecumenical 'prophetic vision' (2001: 32) for the pandemic, for instance, suggests a 'comprehensive' whole-person approach that does not distinguish prevention from treatment, and that also addresses aspects of Mbeki's statements that 'poverty causes HIV'. The solution to the dispute above also involved integration. Like the interviewees in our HIV support research, it took people with HIV as being, despite their specific health and other concerns, 'just like anybody', concerned about childcare, education and employment, and trying, like Yoliswa at the beginning of this chapter, to formulate futures for themselves and their children. And it assumed that people not yet directly affected by HIV – like many of the original playgroup organisers – could understand the different, specific requirements of people living with the virus.

Some neighbourhoods in South Africa have local organisations with long histories of managing conflicts of interest like those involved in the dispute described. Other, newer areas, like many of those where we did the research, rely much more on recent local organisations like the one that mediated the dispute, or on political education, the 'conscientising' and 'responsibilising' (Robins, 2004) performed by organisations such as TAC within local communities. In neither case, given the large but uncertain future of the epidemic, can a theory of how to respond usefully be applied, except at the level of principles of inclusion, democracy, accountability and encouraging community action. The 'local' may be 'global' in some ways, and useful alliances can be constructed across spatial and other sites, but the specific circumstances of neighbourhoods affected by HIV have to be addressed each time, from within.

Personal storytelling styles relate in intimate and interesting ways to public negotiations of the epidemic like those considered above. Attention to personal narrative styles can suggest how ways of talking about and acting within the epidemic are developing, at the level of local citizenship. Addressing personal narratives may also allow difficulties of HIV experiences to be expressed within the fluid structure of people's stories. As people live through ongoing waves of illness and deaths, the importance grows of being able to speak about almost unspeakable things, and of continuing to represent those people pushed into the past by the onrushing present.

In this research on HIV support, intimate disclosure stories, religious, political and other forms of narrative, coexisted in varying balances in the interviewees' accounts. Interviewees' stories presented a set of local, pragmatic theories about how to achieve HIV ownership in widening circles of interpretive community. Such ownership seemed to be an important goal, and acceptance, disclosure and a broader 'speaking out' were important parts of progress towards it. Developing the effective uses of HIV representations was, and remains, difficult. But this research provides many powerful examples of people finding ways to speak about and live with HIV that sustain them, and that comfort, educate and inspire others.

I hope that this book may be helpful in thinking about the strategies which people infected and affected by HIV develop, how these strategies are significant to them, and how they may also be valuable for HIV education, treatment and policy. Emerging from 'gatherings of human beings concerned about turning around one of the greatest threats humankind has faced', as Nelson Mandela put it – in this case support groups, activist campaigns, family interactions, friendship networks and neighbourhood discussions – such strategies are theories in themselves, often the first theories of complex, new phenomena. They are exemplars of pragmatic 'theories' in action.

Notes

Introduction: The many epidemics of HIV

1 Other national and worldwide data cited in the chapter also come from UNAIDS (2006) and UNAIDS/WHO (2006).

2 UK deaths from HIV have stayed relatively constant over the past few years at around 400–500 (Health Protection Agency, 2006).

3 Pragmatism is sometimes regarded as largely antithetical to postmodernism in its implications for citizenship (Hickman, 2004) but the writers drawn on here relate it fruitfully to 'postmodern' and deconstructionist theoretical debates.

4 Some development theorists argue the lack of power of such regional governance within the world system (Hardt and Negri, 2001; Wallerstein, 2004), and on this account have been criticised from an array of positions that point out a variety of simplifications, including the development of Southern alliances, divisions and competition within the Northern bloc, and the power of factors other than the macroeconomic and macropolitical – for instance the microeconomic, political, cultural, nation-state, local state and popular movements. See for instance Skocpol, 1994, and from a South African perspective, the *African Renaissance* collection Makgoba (1999) and Mbembe (2001).

5 Social inclusion and exclusion have been contested categories, most often because they do not necessarily imply social justice (Gray, 2000; Lister, 2000). I use them in the book in accordance with their currency within many debates on HIV policy rather than to denote a theoretical adherence to them.

6 The estimate is low and is epidemiologically driven, drawing on UNAIDS's (2005) most optimistic future scenario of HIV deaths rising till 2013 and prevalence falling to present levels by 2025. A much higher figure could be arrived at by taking less optimistic epidemiological scenarios, factoring in the so far underexplored social effects of HIV on the next generation in high prevalence countries and communities – as indeed these scenarios also do – and considering HIV's likely epidemic continuance at high levels.

7 Poverty is another contested term, not only in its definition but in its usefulness. I continue to use it, again, because of its currency in popular HIV debates within and outside South Africa.

8 Useful overviews of the effects of HIV in South Africa appear in Anarfi (2003), Barnett and Whiteside (2006), Iliffe (2006), Poku and Whiteside (2004) and Whiteside and Sunter (2000). South African life expectancy quoted here comes from Moodley (2006) and a private sector study, but other studies have estimated it at 45.

9 On the early days of Gay Men's Health Crisis, see Kayal (1993). On ACT UP, see Crimp (1988) and ACT UP New York/Women and AIDS Book Group (1990). On

TAC, see Mbali (2005) and Robins (2004); on TASO, see Kaleeba *et al.* (1997). Iliffe (2006, chapter 10) provides an excellent overview of achievements and limitations.

10   These countries' HIV responses are summarised in the UNAIDS (2006) report. Other useful sources are the Avert website at http://www.avert.org and the US Centers for Disease Control website http://www.cdc.gov/nchstp/od/gap/countries/ – accessed 31 July 2006.

11   See also World Health Organisation, 2006a. In international NGOs these medications are often referred to also as ARTs, and in the developed world they have earlier been named combination therapy or 'HAART' (highly active antiretroviral therapy), but 'ARV' was the commonest term used by our research participants in 2001–4.

12   This is particularly salient in the light of continuing high rates of TB worldwide and increasing attention to its multi-drug-resistant and extensive drug-resistant strains. Farmer (1999) analyses waves of developed-world attention to TB in his chapter entitled 'Emerging from where?' See also Gandy and Zumla (2003).

13   Recent research suggests a substantial role of loveLife in young people's lives (Reproductive Health Research Unit/loveLife, 2004). Khomanani evaluations have also indicated some behavioural effects (Health and Development Africa, 2007).

14   Patton (1994) and Richardson (1987) as well as, in the Haitian context, Farmer (1999) provide good summaries.

15   These benefits are R780 monthly. Foster care grants are lower, at R560. Child support is an increasingly taken-up, significant but smaller-scale benefit. Relatively few are eligible for unemployment benefit.

16   Yearly prevalence figures collected from public antenatal clinics do not use these categories, and these clinics tend disproportionately to serve black African women. Coloured/mixed race people constitute 8.8 per cent of the population and Indian/Asian people 2.5 per cent – for population statistics see Statistics South Africa (2001).

17   Estimates vary: Solidarity Peace Trust's (2004) estimate was 1.7 million, refugee organisations' estimates now reach 4 million (South African Broadcasting Corporation, 2006).

18   The National Institutes of Health (2007) for instance are investigating microbicides as HIV and other STI transmission preventers across seven African and 13 other countries.

1 HIV in South Africa: global, local and historical realities

1   A full account from the van der Maas's own perspective is available online at their Power to the People website http://www.powertothepeople.co.za/, accessed 20 October 2006.

2   Immunisation rates are also similar to those of low-income Tanzania (Unicef/World Health Organisations 2006), though infant mortality is lower, largely due to less mortality from malaria.

3   The apartheid regime deliberately destabilised countries throughout southern Africa militarily, politically and economically (Johnson and Martin, 1990). South Africa was, of course, most directly and comprehensively affected by the regime.

4   This account draws on the Aegis AIDS timeline http://www.aegis.com/topics/timeline/default.asp, Avert's HIV history online at http://www.avert.org/historyi.htm, Barnett and Whiteside (2006) and Iliffe (2006).

5   The order of the latter two is disputed; however, see Johnson and Pape (1989).

6   I am using 'mythology' here in a Barthesian (1993) [1957] sense, to indicate a realm of assumed meaning, rather than to indicate a level of fantasy beneath which rests the truth.

7 Injected contraceptives, around six times as frequently provided as oral contraceptives in the area I was researching, and the WHO-trialled anti-fertility 'vaccine' serve at times as supporting evidence.

8 This recalls Selikow *et al.*'s (2002) finding that it is often easier not to have sex than to use condoms.

9 Such impacts are not necessarily helpfully characterised as trauma: see Leys, 2000; Reeler, 1998.

10 See Burns, 2002; Morrell *et al.*, 2002.

11 Rates of child abuse in other countries are also generally high (Andrews *et al.*, 2004; United Nations, 2006). The rape and abuse of young children may be viewed, as with some preferential employment of young sex workers, as a way of minimising HIV risk, or may simply be a form of child abuse not related to HIV (Jewkes, 2004).

12 Robins (2004) suggests considerable continuing hostility to migrants from other African countries within South Africa and some tendency to blame them for the HIV epidemic. See also Harris (2002).

13 Substantial commentary exists on high profile cases so I will only briefly review them here.

14 This history comes largely from Heywood (2005) and Mbali (2003, 2005). See also Philips (2001) on the related histories of this and other South African epidemics.

15 The earlier AIDS Consortium was viewed by some as too gay-oriented.

16 For a mainstream account of GEAR, see the Government of South Africa's (1996) account. For criticisms, see Desai (2002); Gumede (2005); Hart, 2002; Naidoo and Veriava (2003). Under pressure and in the face of growing inequalities, GEAR was dropped in 2002.

17 See Office of the Public Protector Report No. 1 (1996), and Meares (1996).

18 Mbeki is quoted in a *Sunday Times* article (Kortjaas and Msomi, 1998).

19 For research on MTCT efficacy see Connor *et al.* (1994) – reporting a two-thirds reduction in US infant HIV positivity – and Moodley *et al.* (2000) on effective $2 MTCT in South Africa.

20 This followed the Beyond Awareness campaign, still archived online at http://www.cadre.org.za/awareness.htm.

21 Wilbraham (2004); see also Burns (2002) on this sexualisation as a more general tendency and Coulson's (2002) comparative report.

22 Sex researchers and educators can at least help with HIV in South Africa by removing the associations of HIV with guilt and danger, Burns (2002) suggests.

23 Each series is based in literature review, developed and piloted with relevant organisations, and evaluated: see Soul City/MarkData (2005) and Papa *et al.*, (2001); Scheepers *et al.* (2004); Singhal *et al.* (2002) for evaluations.

24 Cameron (2005a, b) – not out about his status despite a 1986 diagnosis – had an activist history of fighting homophobia, and of opposing racism in gay organisations, and fought legal battles for confidentiality around AIDS in the 1990s (Mbali, 2005).

25 In 1997, amid considerable excitement and desperation in the local HIV community, Mbeki had brought a group of South African researchers to talk to the Cabinet about Virodene, a substance with anecdotally reported benefits to the health of people living with HIV. Not only was this substance cheap and apparently effective, it was also, like Kemron, the low-dose alpha-interferon drug developed in Nairobi seven years earlier and announced as an AIDS cure by Kenyan President Daniel Arap Moi, an African solution to an African problem. Kemron showed no clinical effectivity against HIV. Neither did any of the non-ARV chemical substances investigated or sold in the US and Europe as HIV cures during the 1980s

and early 1990s, when no effective conventional treatment was available. Virodene was finally dismissed by the South African Medical Research Council – chaired by Professor Malegapuru Makgoba. In addition to the other histories referenced, see Mbeki (1998) at http://www.anc.org.za/ancdocs/history/mbeki/1998/virodene. html and Aidsmap at http://www.aidsmap-com/cms1632473.asp. Accessed 10 May 2007.

26   Heywood (2005) suggests he was affected in this by Virodene's failure to withstand investigation.

27   Mbeki compared Duesberg to Galileo; his apparent new thinking on HIV earned him the same comparison within the ANC. Cohen (2000a) usefully summarises the argument.

28   This concern was notoriously expressed by a Mbeki spokesperson, Parks Mankahlana, to *Science* magazine (Cohen, 2000b).

29   To which he was urged by Makgoba, at that time President of the Medical Research Council, Cameron, and the Congress of South Africa Trades Unions, COSATU (Heywood, 2005).

30   One informant – interviewed during pilot work, shortly before Johnson's death, and so not reported on in our main study – suggested that Johnson was less ill than he appeared. The interviewee, very ill himself, and involved in an HIV organisation that was at this point close to the government's position, had read the report in the respected *Sowetan* newspaper – in which a reflexologist alleged Johnson was well and being manipulated for money by his white foster mother – and thought there might be something in it (*New York Times*, 2 June 2001).

31   TAC named a branch after Moraka in 2004.

32   Govender (2006) suggests that legal actions are increasingly the only redress in a situation of ANC political domination but powerful constitutional guarantee, and points to the court decision over MTCT as an example. The long-term cooperation of TAC and the AIDS Law Project supports this analysis, but also suggests that such legal actions are driven by grassroots political action. The idea that TAC is led by its professionalised successes is simplistic.

33   The final 2002 judgement again found against the government.

34   Naimak (2006) is a useful description of these programmes as they are developing, as are other papers on the UCT Centre for Social Science Research website.

35   This did not hold if CD4 counts were below 50 (Department of Health, 2004). Earlier MSF guidelines differed. MSF's (Médecins sans Frontières and World Health Organisation, 2003) early project report stated most deaths on ARVs happened early, due to very ill patients starting treatment.

36   Overall in this programme, 55 per cent started with CD4 counts less than 50, with 14 per cent dying in the first two years (Coetzee *et al.*, 2004). See also Abdullah *et al.*, (2006).

37   It is, however, not uncommon within recent ANC discourse including that of Mbeki; see Gumede, 2005.

38   This denialism can be related to Lysenkoism, both in its structures of argument (Geffen, 2006) and, historically, in many senior ANC figures' professional and political formation within the Soviet Union.

39   These programmes, adopted by some traditionalist groups, including women's groups, predominantly in KwaZulu-Natal and the Eastern Cape, draw on historical regulatory practices – but also recall the virginity-sustaining programmes of the early AIDS era in the US, such as 'True Love Waits', despite these earlier programmes' Christian and apparently dual-gender approach, social and personal rather than physical policing. In South Africa virginity testing is also said to be a

weapon against rape and child abuse. See Kiguwa (2004), Leclerc-Madlala (2001) and Morrell *et al.* (2002) for criticisms.

40 Social capital is also an idea whose time has come for the World Bank, as its 'Social Capital for Development' web pages – which do not reference Bourdieu – indicate: http://www1.worldbank.org/prem/poverty/scapital/index.htm.

41 Such actions are in Haiti more strongly and directly related to developed-world activism and resources than in the South African case.

2 Researching HIV

1 This realm spans the stylistically and politically diverse work of, for instance, Gilbert and George, Kiki Smith, Robert Mapplethorpe and Nicholas Nixon.

2 See Aronowitz, 1995; Boffin and Gupta, 1991; Carter and Watney, 1989; Crimp, 1988; Crimp and Ralston, 1990; Murphy and Poirier, 1993; Oppenheimer and Reckitt, 1997; Patton, 1991; Plummer, 1995; Watney, 1991, 1994; Weeks, 1995 for examples.

3 Idol Pictures'1999 and subsequent *Beat It* documentary education series and their TAC-focused 2001 *A Luta Continua* are other prominent South African televisual examples.

4 On the Botswana programme, see Galavotti *et al.* (2001). On the first, 2003, Kenya conference on African soap operas now taking on HIV issues, see Population Communication International, 2003. The CDC initiative in Zimbabwe, *Mopani Junction*, with a listenership estimated at half the population, was closed by the Department of Information and Publicity in 2003, against the wishes of the Department of Health, because it was feared it would have *too much* effect on rural populations; in the process of addressing HIV it was also situating them in 'day-to-day social scenarios' – presumably of rural poverty – that the government found misleading (Zimbabwe *Standard*, 28 July 2003).

5 Listed second behind *Soul City* productions (Soul City/MarkData 2005).

6 McCullen's Cold Heaven exhibit can be viewed on the Christian Aid web-site: http://www.christian-aid.org.uk/news/gallery/dmcullin/09image.html. Gideon Mendel's work appears in Carballera (2003) and on the *Guardian* website – for instance, his project on Mozambiquan HIV orphans is online at http://www.guardian.co.uk/aids/thechildrenleftbehind/gallery/gallery_2.html and at many charity and NGO websites including that of TAC.

7 See the pieces by Ximba, Ximba and Sithole shown at the Siyazama site: http://www.sanch.org/amagugu2/KateWells.htm.

8 Afropop (at http://www.afropop.org/multi/feature/ID/56) features Angelina Kidjo, Baba Maal and Femi Kuti discussing the issue. A Zimbabwean discussion, however, suggests most popular songs on the topic are either mourning or blaming: http://www.rixc.lv/pipermail/xchange/2004-June/000354.html. The 2006 trial of Simon Bikindi, a Rwandan musician accused of using his songs to incite the genocide, points to the dangers of overoptimism about this medium. See also Iliffe, 2006: 81–2.

9 See Note 6.

10 Debates about the exact meaning of social capital are numerous: Bourdieu's (1986) formalist categorisation is more descriptive than Putnam's instrumentalist social ethics. The term is frequently used as a heuristic for community development. Its analogy with economic capital is tangential in Putnam, and can seem by turns reductive and imprecise in Bourdieu.

11 I have referenced here only the first in an influential series.

12 On researching 'others' and from outside see Ratele (2004).

13 Van Valenderen and Neves (2004) argue that despite such problems, PAR still provides a worthwhile framing for research.

14 Cornell (1992) suggests that 'community' itself can be and sometimes is used within such a critical frame. Bourdieu (1986) discusses neighbour relations but only as forms of social capital.

15 This insight is also well-established within PAR.

16 The South African journal *Agenda* has a long history of considering this issue, in for instance its 2001 'African Feminisms' issues 50 and 51. The journal *Feminist Africa* is a more recent resource.

17 This applies to all women under 16 and to non-consenting young women over 16.

18 Gillian Hart's (2002) application of the concept of 'relational generality', focused specifically on South Africa, is relevant here.

19 Many black Africans living in the Western Cape have family connections and land in the Eastern Cape, an area where Xhosa people have historically lived, but to which many were also forcibly displaced in the nineteenth century and later by the apartheid government which constituted parts of it as their 'homeland'.

20 Approval from my employing university's ethics committee in the UK had also been obtained.

21 Demographics forms did not address socioeconomic status but many interviewees mentioned education level while describing their HIV histories.

22 Consent forms were available in Xhosa and English, and discussed with myself and the research assistants in English and the research assistants in Xhosa.

3 Talking about the big thing

1 World Health Organisation (2005) HIV illness definitions for Africa also use weight change guidelines.

2 Stenson *et al.* (2005) found high medical professional and counsellor satisfaction when these staff were able to give counselling about ARVs.

3 In a few cases, generalist clinics had close associations with HIV specialist programmes whose expertise and understanding had been passed on.

4 Several MTCT research participants had younger untested babies or did not discuss the results during interview.

5 These issues were declared resolved in the Western Cape by 2004 (Naimak, 2006).

6 Since this time, donations of e'pap fortified porridge, a version of the traditional South African staple maize meal porridge, from charities and churches, have become widespread, but are not guaranteed provision for HIV positive people.

7 MSF and WHO awareness of the significance of people's treatment involvement rather than simply readiness, points to similar factors (Médecins sans Frontières and World Health Organisation, 2003).

8 For a continent overview of traditional practices in relation to HIV, see Iliffe, 2006: 90ff.

9 Olley *et al.* (2005) also found poor recall of counselling.

10 Skogmar *et al.* (2006) found no association between counselling and disclosure although the nature and understanding of the former could, as here, be variable.

11 In the US, Walch *et al.* (2006) find higher socioeconomic status HIV positive people less willing to use groups; this tended to be true of our very few middle-class interviewees.

12 This is similarly reported in the aftermaths of other traumatic events, for instance, by women survivors of Rwandan genocide and rape (Mukamana and Collins, 2006).

13 Counselling and groups may not be disclosure-significant in the longer-term (Skomar *et al.*, 2006); many of our interviewees were recently diagnosed.

14 In this case, however, 'friends and elders' advising Busisiwe to go back to the city in search of treatment also had the effect of getting this stigmatised person to leave the area.

15 Greene and Faulkner (2002) also point to gossip as a difficult element in women's disclosure decisions, to expectations shaping disclosure, and to the positive support and mental health effects of disclosure for many women.

16 Effective medical treatment may itself be interpreted as a 'miracle', as Farmer (1999) has described happening in Haiti, where TB treatment was so scarce, its effectiveness was not generally known.

17 Rape survivors of the Rwandan genocide who have had children as a result similarly describe the events as 'God's will' (Mukamana and Collins, 2006).

18 The most apposite text here may be Psalm 91.

19 TASO in Uganda and the early transnational concerns of the International Community of Women Living with AIDS are examples.

4 From othering to owning: speaking out about HIV

1 Many thanks to René Brandt for her comments on this chapter.

2 My definition of narrative includes temporal and/or causal succession and requires some – not necessarily personal – particularity (Squire, 2005; forthcoming; Todorov, 1990). While sometimes, entire interviews are legitimately explained as narratives (Riessman, 1993), this book describes interview talk generally in other ways, for instance, as accounts, in order to point to the non-narrative aspects that can also be important within interview talk.

3 For alternative possible approaches to these data, see Squire, forthcoming.

4 Other problems with a genre analysis of this material are addressed in Squire, forthcoming.

5 This model develops Marshall's (1950) notion of civil, political and social citizenship.

6 Rose and Novas (2004), Kleinman (1988), Greenhalgh and Horwitz (1998) and Plummer (1995: 174) discuss such narratives in the fields of biological citizenship, illness and HIV, respectively.

7 I am, of course, assuming some authority here to declare what the stories mean – that is, to theorise them – myself, despite claiming to locate the 'theory' in the stories themselves.

8 Stories are not always theory. Often they are simply told for pleasure, or to fill silence. HIV is a pressing condition, but even its seriousness and immediacy can at times support such stories.

9 Lewis Nkosi (1959) writes about Modisane leaving South Africa in the wake of the destruction of Sophiatown, when apartheid silencing became too much for him to bear. Similarly, Mphaphlele describes the othered displacement of exile in Brutus's writings: 'his is the voice crying in the night, endlessly, without consolation' (1962: 242).

10 Wolfe *et al.* (2006) report reduced HIV stigma in Botswana since national ARV rollout.

11 Mkhise (2004). Ratele and Shefer (2002) note their respondents' frequent equation of sexual repressiveness with 'culture'.

12 Plummer (1995) describes this trajectory well, in relation, for instance, to 'coming out' stories. Earlier empirical research on stories of gay identity formation relate similar progresses (Cass, 1979; Troiden, 1979). However, Plummer's (1995) account is also more general, taking in stories around rape, sexual harassment and abuse, and feminist consciousness-raising.

13 The Xhosa word generally translated as 'shock' has connotations of being physically checked, as indeed the word has in English.

14 Afrikaans speakers may also call HIV 'that thing' (Uys, 2002: 154–5).

15 Dowling (n.d.) discusses metaphor and HIV in Xhosa. Similar indirection can also be found in non-African languages. See also Guzuna (2000) on women and Xhosa.

16 We analysed all self-references to come to this conclusion.
17 Indeed, Olley *et al.* (2005) find significant levels of PTSD directly attributable to the diagnosis and associated with depression, suicidal thinking, work impairment and alcohol abuse.
18 Although the facilitator's 'instructive' knowledge is foregrounded in this account, it was clear in all accounts of groups that facilitators were not prescriptive.
19 The dialogue layout was introduced by the transcriber to represent reported speech.
20 In Thailand, support group membership has been found to relate to treatment access (Vanlandingham *et al.*, 2006).
21 Dowling (n.d) says playfulness equates with not taking things seriously in African languages. However, Busisiwe's carefully judged 'humorous' stories, told 'as if I am joking', are clearly serious.
22 In particular, Ahmed's (2004) account of feelings as metonymically produced by the chaining of signifiers is relevant here; see also Squire, 2006.
23 Kristeva is often criticised for a maternocentrism ultimately under control of a phallocentric Law. Nevertheless, her formulation of the abject comes close to the quality of people's HIV representations (Williamson, 1989; see also Gross, 1990).
24 This is also the case for stigma, which is perhaps grounded in abjection.
25 I shall not discuss the abjectification of 'transgressive' non-heterosexual sexualities here. Interviewees did not mention gay and lesbian sexualities specifically in relation to HIV, although some of their references to HIV as a western disease and to transgressive sexualities seemed to connote them.

5 Living positively: religious and moral narratives of HIV

1 I would like to thank Anthea Williams for her valuable help with this chapter's engagement with religious texts.
2 Augustine's *Confessions* are an often-cited beginning of this tradition, but the linking of personal rebirth to a belief event is more definitive of later texts. Shea (1968) usefully describes both the variability and the conventionalism of canonic Puritan spiritual autobiography.
3 The criteria mentioned here are also used in Squire 1999 and 2003. However, some narrative researchers are prepared to describe genres arising from their body of data *sui generis* (no pun intended) and justify this by referring to the validity of their data and the robustness of their interpretation.
4 I am indebted to Lumka Daniel for her insight on this.
5 Krog (2000) notes that TRC translators drew on the language of the King James Bible as the most appropriate resource to deal with some complexly spoken Xhosa testimony.
6 Mphaphlele (1962) discusses religious discourse's collusions with colonialism as well as its emancipatory use by African writers.
7 http://www.cuaha.info/index2.php. This website (accessed 20 September 2006) describes the organisation's activities.
8 Accessed 20 September 2006: http://www.christian-aid.org.uk/news/media/press rel/060321p.htm. See also Akinfe, 2006.
9 Farmer (1999) notes a similar move within the Haitian epidemic.
10 There are groups of gay Anglicans in Africa, gay Islamic groups all over the world and some large lesbian and gay evangelical protestant churches in the US.
11 *Soul* magazine, Letters, February/March 2006, p4: from Kbensani Motsi.
12 In John 8: 32, Jesus says, 'You will know the truth, and the truth will set you free'.
13 Corinthians 2: 8. The response here is to trust in God's grace as the believer's infirmities are precious to Him, and indeed to 'glory in my infirmities'.
14 This interview segment mixed English, Afrikaans and Xhosa and is therefore presented also below.

Busisiwe: Yes, because church is very important because I can't stay there and say 'please God help me.' Net three years I can tell another people with something HIV positive see me there jy ken nie for myne se goete. Iya I stay here talk net for ukuba ndithethe ngoba otherwise ndizozama from my friends.

15 Isaiah 40: 4, King James; the protection of the faithful is described in Chapter 1.
16 Such interconnections also characterise religious writing generally, including its addresses to the epidemic (Mahlangu-Ngcobo, 2001).
17 This account is analysed more briefly in Squire, forthcoming.
18 This negotiation is explored further in Squire, forthcoming.
19 Nongqause was also invoked in this vein in Mbeki's 'I am an African' speech on the occasion of the adoption of the new Constitution.

6 Talking politics

1 West (1989) suggests that Foucault's account of the constitution of political subjects runs the risk of reducing politics to subjecthood. However, in this chapter I am primarily concerned with such subjecthood.
2 Mbali (2005) suggests the usefulness of rights arguments in certain developing-world contexts such as the South African HIV epidemic, despite their theoretical and policy limitations.
3 Gumede (2005) gives a thorough, recent and accessible account of these heterogeneities.
4 Tarrow (2005: 186) emphasises the pre-existence of mobilisation on all involved countries as a condition for successful transnational activism.
5 Much of such effective writing, which also addressed identities and ethics, was, though, fictional (Ndebele, 1994).
6 Criticisms of the normalisation of gay and lesbian sexualities by familial tropes seem in this context less significant than those tropes' inclusive effects.
7 Koyana is discussing Sindiwe Magona's *To My Children's Children* (1990), addressed to her great-grand-daughter, and other writings.
8 For a recent debate, see *Feminist Africa* (2004), issue 3, online http://www.feministafrica.org/03-2004/index.html accessed 1 November 2006.
9 Online http://www.who.int/hiv/photostories/en/index.html. Accessed 1 November 2006. WHO's previous photostory campaign was more ambivalently entitled 'Stories of Tragedy and Hope'

References

Abdool Karim, S. (1998) Placebo controls in HIV perinatal transmission trials: A South African's viewpoint. *American Journal of Public Health* 88 (4): 566

Abdool Karim, Q. and Abdool Karim, S. (2002) The evolving HIV epidemic in South Africa. *International Journal of Epidemiology* 31: 37–40

Abdool Karim, Q. and Abdool Karim, S. (2005) *HIV/AIDS in South Africa*. Cambridge: Cambridge University Press

Abdullah, F., Besser, M., Naledi, T., Boulle, A., Mazwi, Z., and Shaikh, N. (2002) Upscaling prevention of mother to child transmission programmes in the Western Cape Province of South Africa: Implementation, Early Performance and Operational Challenges. International AIDS Conference, Barcelona, July

Abdullah, F., Bock, P., Osler, M. and Boulle, A. (2006) Clinical Outcomes in ART Scale Up, Western Cape Province of South Africa. International AIDS Conference, Toronto, July

Achmat, Z. (2001) Interview with Zackie Achmat. *Multinational Monitor* 22: 1–2, January–February. Online http://multinationalmonitor.org/mm2001/01jan-feb/interview.html. Accessed 10 August 2006

Achmat, Z. (2006) Make truth powerful: leadership in science prevention and the treatment of HIV/AIDS. Closing address, Microbicides 2006 conference. Online http://www.tig.org.2a/pdf-filesaffadavit-aug06/62A%20at%Microbicides%202006%20conference.pdf. Accessed 1 April 2007

ACTUP New York/Women and AIDS Book Group (1990) *Women, AIDS and Activism*. Boston, MA: South End Press

African Union (2006) Universal Access to HIV/AIDS, Tuberculosis and Malaria Services by 2010. Aide memoire. Abuja: African Union.

Aggleton, P. and Homans, D. (1988) *Social Aspects of AIDS*. Brighton: Falmer Press.

Ahmed, S. (2004) *The Cultural Politics of Emotions*. Edinburgh: Edinburgh University Press

Akinfe, A. (2006) Cast iron curtain. *Positive Nation* 127: 25–6

Amaro, H. (1988) Considerations for prevention of HIV infection among Hispanic women. *Psychology of Women Quarterly* 12: 429–43

Andrews, G. Carry, J., Slade, T., Issakidis, C. and Swanston, H. (2004) Child sexual abuse. In M. Ezzati, A. Lopez, A. Rodgers, and C. Murra (eds) *Comparative Quantification of Health Risks: Global and Regional Burden of Disease Attributable to Selected Risk Factors*. Volume 2. Geneva: World Health Organisation

Anarfi, J. (2003) The impact of HIV/AIDs on Africa. *New Agenda* 9: 33–45

Annan, K. (2004) UN Secretary-General's remarks on International Women's Day, 8 March 2004, New York. Online http://www.un.org/apps/sg/sgstats.asp?nid=806. Accessed 31 July 2006

Armistead, L., Tannenbaum, L., Forehand, R., Morse, E. and Morse, P. (2001) Disclosing HIV status: are mothers telling their children? *Journal of Pediatric Psychology* 26: 11–20

Aronowitz, S. (1995) Against the Liberal State: ACT-UP and the Politics of Pleasure. In L. Nicholson and S. Seidman (eds) *Social Postmodernism: Beyond Identity*. Cambridge: Cambridge University Press

Bakhtin, M. (1986) *Speech Genres and Other Late Essays*. Austin, TX: University of Texas Press

Barnett, A. and Whiteside, A. (2006) *AIDS in the Twenty-First Century*. London: Palgrave Macmillan

Barnett, C. (2004) Yizo Yizo: Citizenship, commodification and popular culture in South Africa. *Media Culture and Society* 26 (2): 251–71

Barthes, R. (1993) [1957] *Mythologies*. London: Vintage

Baylies, C. and Bujra, J. (2001) *AIDS, Sexuality and Gender in Africa: The Struggle Continues*. London: UCL Press

Bermudez Ribiero de la Cruz, B. (2004) From policy to practice: the anthropology of condom use. In K. Kaufman and D. Lindauerf (eds), *AIDS and South Africa: The Social Expression of a Pandemic*. London: Palgrave Macmillan

Bernstein, H. (1978) *No. 46 – Steve Biko*. London: International Defence and Aids Fund

Biko, S. (1996) *I Write What I Like*. London: Bowerdean Publishing

Boffin, T. and Gupta, S. (eds) (1991). *Ecstatic Antibodies*. London: River's Oram Press

Bor, R., Miller, R. and Goldman, E. (1993) *Theory and Practice of HIV Counselling*. New York: Brunner Mazel

Bourdieu, P. (1986). The forms of capital. In J.G. Richardson (ed.) *Handbook of Theory and Research for the Sociology of Education*. New York: Greenwood Press

Brandt, R. (2005) Coping with HIV/AIDS: A case analysis of the experiences of poor, HIV positive mothers and women care givers on HAART. Cape Town: Centre for Social Science Research Working Paper 120

Brecher, J., Costello, T. and Smith, B. (2000) *Globalization From Below*. Boston, MA: South End Press

Burns, C. (2002) A commentary on the colloquium Instituting Gender Equality in Schools: Working in an HIV/AIDS Environment. *Agenda* 53: 6–10

Bury, M. (1982) Chronic illness as biographical disruption. *Sociology of Health and Illness* 4 (2): 167–82

Bury, M. (2001) Illness narratives, fact or fiction? *Sociology of Health and Illness* 21 (3): 263–85

Butchart, A. (1998) *The Anatomy of Power: European Constructions of the African Body*. London: Zed Press

Butler, J. (1993) *Bodies that Matter*. London: Routledge

Cameron, E. (2005a) *Witness to AIDS*. London: IB Tauris

Cameron, E. (2005b) Interview. *Positive Nation* 115: 25–6

Campbell, C. (2003) *Letting them Die? Why HIV/AIDS Prevention Programmes Fail*. Oxford: James Currey

Campbell, C., Foulis, C., Maimarn, S. and Sibuya, Z. (2005) The impact of social environments on the effectiveness of youth HIV prevention: A South African case study. *AIDS Care* 17(4): 471–8

Carballeira, P. (2003) *A Broken Landscape*. London: Blume

Carricaburu, D. and Pierret, J. (1995) From biographical disruption to biographical reinforcement: the case of HIV and men. *Sociology of Health and Illness* 17: 65–88

Carter, E. and Watney, S. (1989) *Taking Liberties*. London: Serpent's Tail

Cass, V. (1979) Homosexual identity formation: a theoretical model. *Journal of Homosexuality* 4: 219–35

Centers for Disease Control (2004) *Cases of HIV Infection and AIDS in the United States, 2004*. Online http://www.cdc.gov/hiv/topics/surveillance/resources/reports/index.htm. Accessed 10 October 2006

Centre for the Study of Violence and Reconciliation and Khulamani Support Group n.d.). Survivors' perceptions of the Truth and Reconciliation Commission and suggestions for the final report. Online http://www.csvr.org.za/papers/papkhul.htm. Accessed 1 November 2006

Charlesworth, H. (2005) Not waving but drowning: Gender mainstreaming and human rights in the United Nations. *Harvard Human Rights Journal* 18: 3–18

Cherian, L. (2004) Influence of culture and religion in HIV/AIDS education in South Africa. International AIDS Conference, Bangkok, July

Chirimuuta, R. and Chirimuuta, R. (1989) *AIDS, Africa and Racism*. London: Free Association Books

Ciambrone, D. (2001) Illness and other assaults on self: The relative impacts of HIV/AIDS on women's lives. *Sociology of Health and Illness* 23: 517–40

Clark. S. (2004) Early marriage and HIV risks in sub-Saharan Africa. *Studies in Family Planning* 35(3) September: 149–60

Clark, J. (2006) Discourses of Transition in South Africa. PhD Thesis, Manchester Metropolitan University.

Coetzee D., Hildebrand, K., Boulle, A., Maartens, G., Louis, F., Labatala, V., Reuter, H., Ntwana, N. and Goemaere, E. (2004) Outcomes after two years of providing antiretroviral treatment in Khayelitsha, South Africa. *AIDS* 18: 887–95

Cohen, J. (2000a) South Africa AIDS Researchers Decry Mbeki's Views on HIV. *Science* Vol. 288, No. 5466: 590–1

Cohen, J. (2000b) South Africa's new enemy. *Science* Vol. 288, No. 5474: 2168–70

Cohen, Judah (2004) To sing of AIDS in Uganda. Doctors for Global Health, 2004. Online http://www.dghonline.org/nl14/uganda_music.html. Accessed 20 August 2006

Connor, E.M., Sperling, R.S., Gelber, R. (1994) Reduction of maternal-infant transmission of human immunodeficiency virus type 1 with zidovudine treatment. *New England Journal of Medicine* 331: 1173–80

Cook, R. (1994) *Human Rights of Women: National and International Perspectives*. Philadelphia, PA: University of Pennsylvania Press

Coppa, K. and Boyle, F. (2003). The role of self-help groups in chronic illness management. *Australian Journal of Primary Health* 9 (2 & 3): 68–74

Corliss, R. (1994) The Gay Gauntlet. Now that Philadelphia is a hit, can Hollywood still shun gay themes? *Time* 143(6), 7 February

Cornell, D. (1992) *The Philosophy of the Limit*. New York: Routledge

Cornish, F. (2004) Making 'context' concrete: a dialogical approach to the society–health relation. *Journal of Health Psychology* 9: 281–94

Corti, L., Day, A. and Backhouse, G. (2000) Confidentiality and informed consent: Issues for consideration in the preservation of and provision of access to qualitative data archives. *Forum Qualitative Sozialforschung / Forum: Qualitative Social Research* 1 (3). Online http://www.qualitative-research.net/fqs-texte/3–00/3–00 cortietal-e.htm. Accessed 1 November 2006

COSATU (2005) *Proposal, People's Budget*. Johannesburg: Naledi Press

Coulson, N. (2000) Developments in the use of the mass media at the national level for HIV/AIDS prevention in South Africa. The Communication Initiative. Online http://www.comminit.com/strategicthinking/stcoulson/sld-1541.html. Accessed 10 October 2006

Coward, R. (1989) *The Whole Truth*. London: Faber & Faber

Craib, I. (1994) *The Importance of Disappointment*. London: Routledge

Craib, I. (2004) Telling stories. In M. Andrews, S.D. Sclater, C. Squire and A. Treacher (eds) *The Uses of Narrative*. New Jersey: Continuum

Crimp, D. (1988) *AIDS: Cultural Analysis/Cultural Activism*. Boston, MA: MIT Press

Crimp, D. and Ralston, A. (1990) *AIDS Demo/Graphics*. Seattle, WA: Bay Press

Crossley, M. (2000) *Introducing Narrative Psychology: Self, Trauma and the Construction of Meaning*. Buckingham: Open University Press

Davison, K., Pennebaker, J. and Dickerson, S. (2000) Who talks? The social psychology of illness support groups. *American Psychologist* 55: 205–17

De Man, P. (1983) *The Rhetoric of Romanticism*. New York: Columbia University Press

Denzin, N. (1993) *The Alcoholic Society*. New Brunswick, NJ: Transaction

Department of Health (1998) Press release issued by the Department of Health on the killing of Ms Gugu Dlamini (AIDS case worker). Online http://www.info.gov.za/speeches/1998/990428438p1006.htm. Accessed 1 November 2006

Department of Health (2004) *National Antiretroviral Treatment Guidelines*. Pretoria : Department of Health. Online http://www.doh.gov.za/docs/factsheets/guidelines/artguidelines04/i0africa%22. Accessed 20 August 2006

Department of Health (2005a) *National HIV and Syphilis Ante-natal Sero-Prevalence Survey in South Africa, 2004*. Pretoria: Department of Health. Online http://www.doh.gov.za/docs/reports/2004/hiv-syphilis.pdf. Accessed 20 August 2006

Department of Health (2005b) *Declaration of Commitment on HIV and AIDS*. Online http://www.doh.gov.za/docs/reports/2006/ungass/index.html. Accessed 31 July 2006

Department of Health (2006) *National HIV and Syphilis Ante-natal Sero-Prevalence Survey in South Africa, 2005*. Pretoria: Department of Health. Online http://www.doh.gov.za/docs/reports/2005/hiv-syphilis.pdf. Accessed 20 August 2006

Department of Health (2007) HIV and AIDS and STI Strategic Plan for South Africa, 2007–11. Online http://www.doh.gov.2a/docs/misc/stratplan-f.html. Accessed 10 May 2007

Derrida, J. (1992) The law of genre. In D. Attridge (ed.) *Acts of Literature*. London: Routledge

Derrida, J. (1995) *The Gift of Death*. Chicago: Chicago University Press

Desai, A. (2002) *We are the Poors*. New York: Monthly Review Press

Dowling, T. (n.d.) HIV/AIDS and African Languages. Cape Town: African Voices. Online http://www.africanvoices.co.za/. Accessed 20 August 2006

Dunkle, K., Jewkes, R., Brown, H., Gray, G., Mcintyre, J. and Harlow, S. (2004) Transactional sex among women in Soweto, South Africa: Prevalence, risk factors and association with HIV infection. *Social Science & Medicine*, 59 (8): 1581–92

Edelstein, J. (2002) *Truth and Lies: Stories from the Truth and Reconciliation Commission in South Africa*. New York: New Press.

Edwards, B. and Foley, M. (1998) Civil society and social capital beyond Putnam. *American Behavioral Scientist* 42: 124–39

Elliot, A. (2006) A head full of snakes. *Positive Nation* 127: 37–8

Elsey, H., Tolhurst, R. and Theobald, S. (2005) Mainstreaming HIV/AIDS in development sectors: Have we learned the lessons from gender mainstreaming? *AIDS Care* 17 (8): 988–98

Ezzy, D. (2000) Illness narrative: time, hope and HIV. *Social Science and Medicine* 50: 605–17

Fanon, F. (1986) *Black Skin, White Masks*. London: Pluto

Farmer, P. (1999) *Infections and Inequalities*. Berkeley, CA: University of California Press

Favot, I., Ngalula, J., Mgala, A., Klokke, A., Gumodoka, B. and Boerma, J. (1997) HIV infection and sexual behaviour among women with infertility in Tanzania: A hospital-based study. *International Journal of Epidemiology* 26 (2): 414–19

Fawzi, W., Gernard, I., Msamanga, M. *et al.* (2004) A randomized trial of multivitamin supplements and HIV disease progression and mortality. *New England Journal of Medicine* 351 (1): 23–32

Foucault, Michel (1979) *History of Sexuality Volume 1*. London: Allen Lane

Foucault, Michel (1988) *The Care of the Self*. New York: Vintage Books

Freud, S. (1925) The Uncanny. In *Standard Edition of the Works of Sigmund Freud*, Vol. 17. London: Hogarth Press and the Institute of Psycho-Analysis

Freund, B. (2006) The state of South Africa's cities. In S. Buhlungu, J. Daniel, R. Southall and J. Lutchman (eds) *State of the Nation: South Africa 2005–6*. Cape Town: HSRC Press

Friedman, S. *et al.* (1981) Followup on Kaposi's Sarcomi and *Pneumocystis* Pneumonia. 409–10 *Morbidity and Mortality Weekly Report* 30 August 28 409–10. Online http://www.cdc.gov/hiv/resources/reports/mmwr/pdf/mmwr28aug81.pdf. Accessed 10 October 2006

Frosh, S. (2002) *After Words*. London: Palgrave Macmillan

Frosh, S., Phoenix, A. and Pattman, R. (2003) *Young Masculinities*. London: Palgrave Macmillan

Gaitskell, D. (1997) Power and prayer in service: Women's Christian organisations. In R. Elphick and R. Davenport (eds) *Christianity in South Africa*. Berkeley and Los Angeles: University of California Press

Galavotti, C., Pappas-DeLuca, K. and Lansky, A. (2001) Modeling and reinforcement to combat HIV: The MARCH approach to behavior change. *American Journal of Public Health* 91, 1602–7

Gandy, M. and Zumla, A. (2003) *The Return of the White Plague*. London: Verso

Geffen, N. (2006) *Echoes of Lysenkoism: State-sponsored Pseudo-Science in South Africa*. CSSR Working Paper 149. Cape Town: University of Cape Town Centre for Social Science Research. Online http://www.tac.org.za/documents/wp149.pdf. Accessed 20 October 2006

Gibson, K. and Schwartz, L. (2004) Community psychology: Emotional processes in political subjects. In D. Hook, N. Mkhise, P. Kiguwa, and A. Collins (eds) *Critical Psychology*. Lansdowne, Western Cape: University of Cape Town Press

Gilbert, D. and Wright, E. (2002) *African American Women and HIV/AIDS: Critical Responses*. New York: Praeger

Gilman, S. (1985) *Difference and Pathology*. Ithaca, NY: Cornell University Press

Glaser, E. and Putnam, L. (1991) *In the Absence of Angels*. New York: Putnam

Gobodo-Madikizela, P. (2003) *A Human Being Died That Night*. Cape Town: David Philip Publishers

Goffman, E. (1960) *Stigma*. Harmondsworth: Penguin

Goodwin, J., Jasper, J. and Pollelta, F. (2001) *Passionate Politics: Emotions and Social Movements*. Chicago: University of Chicago Press

Gouws, A. (2006) The state of the national gender machinery: structural problems and personalised politics. In S. Buhlungu, J. David, R. Southall and J. Lutchman (eds) *State of the Nation: South Africa 2005–6*. Cape Town: HSRC Press.

Goulder, P. and Watkins, D. (2004) HIV and SIV CTL escape: Implications for vaccine design. *National Review of Immunology* 4: 630–40

Govender, K. (2006) Assessing the constitutional protection of human rights in South Africa during the first decade of democracy. In S. Buhlungu, J. Daniel, R. Southall and J. Lutchman (eds) *State of the Nation: South Africa 2005–6*. Cape Town: HSRC Press

Government of South Africa (1996) *Growth, Employment and Redistribution: A Macroeconomic Strategy*. Online http://www.polity.org.za/html/govdocs/policy/growth.html?rebookmark=1. Accessed 10 October 2006

Gray, J. (2000) Inclusion: a radical critique. In P. Askonas and A. Stewart (eds) *Social Inclusion: Possibilities and Tension*. Basingstoke: Macmillan Press

Green, G. (1993) Social support and HIV. *AIDS Care* 5: 87–104

Greene, K. and Faulkner, S. (2002) Expected versus actual responses to disclosure in relationships of HIV-positive African American adolescent females. *Communication Studies* 53(4): 297–317

Greenhalgh, T. and Hurwitz, D. (1998) *Narrative-Based Medicine*. London: BMA Books

Gross, E. (1990) The body of signification. In J. Fletcher and A. Benjamin (eds) *Abjection, Melancholia and Loss*. London: Routledge

Gumede, W. (2005) *Thabo Mbeki and the Battle for the Soul of the ANC*. South Africa: Zebra Press

Guzuna, Z. (2000) Exploring women's silence in isiXhosa written and oral literature. *Agenda* 46: 75–81.

Gysels, M., Pool, R. and Nyanzi, S. (2005) The adventures of the Randy Professor and Angela the Sugar Mummy: Sex in fictional serials in Ugandan popular magazines. *AIDS Care* 17 (8): 967–77

Hall, S. (1992) Cultural studies and its theoretical legacies. In L. Grossberg, C. Nelson and P. Treichler (eds) *Cultural Studies*. New York: Routledge

Hall, S. (1994) Cultural identity and diaspora. In P.Williams and L. Chrisman (eds) *Colonial Discourse and Postcolonial Theory: A Reader*. Hemel Hempstead: Harvester Wheatsheaf

Hardt, M. and Negri, A. (2001) *Empire*. Cambridge, MA: Harvard University Press

Harris, B. (2002) Xenophobia: A new pathology for a new South Africa? In D. Hook, amd G. Eagle (eds) *Psychopathology and Social Prejudice*. Cape Town: University of Cape Town Press

Hart, G. (2002) *Disabling Globalisation: Places of Power in Post-Apartheid South Africa*. Berkeley, CA: University of California Press

Hassim, S. (2004) 'A virtuous circle of representation? Gender equality in South Africa. In J. Daniel, J. Lutchman and R. Southall, R. (eds) *The State of the Nation 2004*. Pretoria: HSRC Press

Hastings, A. (1994) *The Church in Africa: 1450–1950*. Oxford: Clarendon Press

Head, B. (1968) *When Rain Clouds Gather*. New York: Simon & Schuster

Health and Development Africa (2007) *Impact assessment of the Khomanani Campaign*. Parktown South Africa: Health and Development Africa

Health Protection Agency (2005) *Mapping the issues: HIV and other sexually transmitted infections in the UK: 2005*. London: Health Protection Agency Centre for Infections

Heelas, P. and Woodhead, L. (2005) *The Spiritual Revolution: Why Religion is Giving Way to Spirituality*. Oxford, UK and Malden, USA: Blackwell

Heath, Stephen (1982) *The Sexual Fix*. London: Macmillan

Heelas, P. and Woodhead, L. (2005) *The Spiritual Revolution: Why Religion is Giving Way to Spirituality*. Oxford, UK and Malden, USA: Blackwell

Hemson, D. and O'Donovan, M. (2006) Putting numbers to a score-card: presidential targets and the state of delivery. In S. Buhlungu, J. Daniel, R. Southall and J. Lutchman (eds) *State of the Nation: South Africa 2005–06*. Cape Town: HSRC Press

Herek, G. (1990) Illness, stigma, and AIDS. In P. Costa and G.R. VandenBos (eds) *Psychological Aspects of Serious Illness*. Washington, DC: American Psychological Association

Heywood, Mark (2005) The Price of Denial. Online www.tac.org.za/Documents/PriceOfDenial.doc. Accessed 10 August 2006

Hickman, L. (2004) Pragmatism and global citizenship. *Metaphilosophy* 35 (1–2): 26–68

Hindmarsh, B. (2005) *The Evangelical Conversion Narrative: Spiritual Autobiography in Early Modern England*. Oxford: Oxford University Press

Holdstock, T. (2000) *Re-examining Psychology: Critical Perspectives and African Insights*. London: Routledge

Hook, D. (2004) Critical psychology and the psychoanalysis of racism. In D. Hook, N. Mkhise, P. Kiguwa and A. Collins (eds) *Critical Psychology*. Lansdowne, Western Cape: University of Cape Town Press

hooks, b. and West, C. (1991) *Breaking Bread*. Boston, MA: South End Press

Huff, B. (2005) Treat the World. *Positive Nation* 114, August: 20–2

Hutchinson, P. and Mahlalela, X. (2006) Utilisation of voluntary counselling and testing services in the Eastern Cape, South Africa. *AIDS Care* 18 (5): 446–55

Iliffe, J. (2006) *The African AIDS Epidemic: A History*. Athens, OH: Ohio University Press

Inglehart, R. and Norris, P. (2004) *Sacred and Secular: Religion and Politics Worldwide*. Cambridge: Cambridge University Press

Jacobs, A. (2003) What narrative theology forgot. *First Things* 135: *First Things* 135: 25–30, August/September: 25–30. Online http://www.firstthings.com/ftissues/ft 0308/articles/jacobs.html. Accessed 20 September 2006

Jelsma, J., MacLean, E., Hughes, J., Tinise, X. and Darder, M. (2005) An investigation into the health-related quality of life of individuals living with HIV who are receiving HAART. *AIDS Care* 17 (5): 579–88

Jewkes, R. (2004) Child sexual abuse and HIV infection. In A. Dawes, L. Richter and C. Higson-Smith (eds) *Sexual Abuse in Children in South Africa*. Cape Town: HSRC Press

Jewkes, R. and Abrahams, N. (2002) The epidemic of rape and sexual coercion in South Africa: An overview. *Social Science and Medicine* 55: 1231–44

Joffe, H. (1997) The relationship between representationalist and materialist perspectives: AIDS and 'the other'. In L. Yardley (ed.) *Material Discourses of Health and Illness*. London: Routledge

Joffe, H. and Bettega, N. (2003) Social representation of AIDS among Zambian adolescents. *Journal of Health Psychology* 8: 616–31

Johnson, L. and Dorrington, J. (2006) Modelling the demographic impact of HIV/AIDS in South Africa and the likely impact of interventions. *Demographic Research* 14: 541–74. Online http://www.demographic-research.org/volumes/vol14/22/14–22. pdf#search='dorrington%20demographic%20user%20guide. Accessed 10 October 2006

Johnson, N. (2001) Speech at the International AIDS Conference, Durban. Online http://www.nkosi.iafrica.com/contentPage.asp?pageID=7. Accessed 10 October 2006

Johnson, P. and Martin, D. (1990) *Apartheid Terrorism: The Destablisation Report.* Bloomington, IN: Indiana University Press

Johnson, W. and Pape, J. (1989) AIDS in Haiti. *Immunological Review* 44: 65–78

Jones, J. (1972) *Prejudice and Racism.* Reading, MA: Addison Wesley

Jones, J. (1993) *Bad Blood: The Tuskegee Syphilis Experiment.* New York: Free Press.

Jones, S., Sherman, G. and Varga, C. (2005) Exploring socio-economic conditions and poor follow-up rates of HIV-exposed infants in Johannesburg, South Africa. *AIDS Care* 17 (4): 466–70

Kaleeba, N., Kalibala, S., Kaseje, M., Ssebbanja, P., Anderson, S., Van Praag, E., Tembo, G. and Katabira, E. (1997). Participatory evaluation of counselling, medical and social services of the AIDS Support Organisastion (TASO) in Uganda. *AIDS Care* 9 (1): 13–26

Kaufman, K. and Lindauer, D. (2003) *AIDS and South Africa: The Social Expression of a Pandemic.* London: Palgrave Macmillan

Kayal, P. (1993) *Bearing Witness: Gay Men's Health Crisis and the Politics of AIDS.* Boulder, CO: Westview Press

Keele, B. *et al* (2006) Chimpanzee reservoirs of pandemic and non-pandemic HIV-1. *Science*, Vol. 313, No. 5786: 523–6

Kelly, J., St Lawrence, J., Diaz, Y., Stevenson, L., Hauth, A., Brasfield, T., Kalichman, S., Smith, J. and Andrew, M. (1991). HIV risk behavior reduction following intervention with key opinion leaders of a population: An experimental community level analysis. *American Journal of Public Health* 81: 168–71

Kiguwa, P. (2004) Feminist critical psychology in Africa. In D. Hook, N. Mkhise, P. Kiguwa and A. Collins (eds) *Critical Psychology.* Lansdowne, Western Cape: University of Cape Town Press

Kimberly, J.A., Serovich, J.M. and Greene, K. (1995) Disclosure of HIV-positive status: Five women's stories. *Family Relations* 44: 316–22

King, L., Dixon, V. and Nobles, W. (1976) *African Philosophy: Assumptions and Paradigms for Research on Black People.* Los Angeles, CA: Fanon Center Publications

Kingsnorth, P. (2003) *One No, Many Yeses.* London: Simon & Schuster

Kleinman, A. (1988) *The Illness Narratives.* New York: Basic Books

Knowlton, A., Hua, Q.W. and Latkin, C. (2004) Social support among HIV positive injection drug users. *AIDS and Behavior* 8 (4): December: 357–63

Koopman, N. (2005) *Churches, Democracy and the Public Sphere.* Cape Town: South African Council of Churches. Online http://www.sacc-ct.org.za/koopman.html. Accessed 20 September 2006

Kortjaas, B. and Msomi, S. (1998) Mob kills woman for telling truth: Health worker stoned and beaten for confession about HIV. *Sunday Times of South Africa*, 27 December

Kramer, L. (1985) *The Normal Heart. New* York: Grove Press.

Krieger, N., Rowley, D., Herman, A., Avery, B. and Phillips, M. (1993) Racism, sexism and social class: implications for studies of health, disease and well-being

American Journal of Preventive Medicine 9 November–December (Supplement): 82–122

Kristeva. J. (1984) *Powers of Horror*. New York: Columbia University Press

Krog, A. (2000) *In the Country of my Skull*. New York: Vintage

Kushner, T. (1993) *Angels in America*. New York: Theatre Communications Group

Kuzwayo, E. (2004) [1985] *Call Me Woman*. London: Picador

Labov, W. (1997) Some further steps in narrative analysis. *Journal of Narrative and Life History* 7 (1–4): 395–415

Lasch, C. (1991) *The Culture of Narcissism*. New York: Norton

Laubscher, L. (2003) Suicide in a South African town: A cultural-psychological investigation. *South African Journal of Psychology* 33 (3): 133–43

Leclerc-Madlala, S. (2001) Virginity testing: managing sexuality in a maturing AIDS epidemic in South Africa. *Medical Anthropology Quarterly* 15 (4): 533–52

Levin, A. (2005) *Aidsafari*. Cape Town: Zebra Press

Leys, R. (2000) *Trauma: A Geneaology*. Chicago, IL: University of Chicago Press

Lister, R. (2000) Strategies for social inclusion: Promoting social cohesion or social justice? In P. Askonas and A. Stewart (eds) *Social Inclusion: Possibilities and Tensions*. Basingstoke: Macmillan

Lown, E., Winkler, K. Fullilove, R. and Fullilove, M. (1993). Tossin' and tweakin': women's consciousness in the crack culture. In C. Squire (ed.) *Women and AIDS: Psychological Perspectives*. London: Sage.

Lutambi, A. (2005) Demographical evolution of the HIV epidemic in Tanzania and South Africa. Dissertation, African Institute for Mathematical Sciences, Cape Town

Lykes, B., Lykes, M.B., TerreBlanche, M. and Hamber, B. (2003). Narrating survival and change in Guatemala and South Africa: The politics of representation and a liberatory community psychology. *American Journal of Community Psychology* 31 (1–2): 79–90

McGregor, L. (2006) *Khabzela: The Life and Times of a South African*. Pretoria: Jacana Press.

Machel, G. and Cravero, K. (2004) Op-ed, World AIDS Day. Geneva: UNAIDS. Online http://data.unaids.org/Media/Press-Statements01/PS_Cravero-Machel_Op Ed-WAD2004_en.pdf. Accessed 1 November 2006

MacIntyre, A. (1984) *After Virtue*. Bloomington, IN: University of Notre Dame Press

MacLeod, C. (2004) Writing into action: the critical research endeavour. In D. Hook, N. Mkhise, P. Kiguwa and A. Collins (eds) *Critical Psychology*. Lansdowne, Western Cape: University of Cape Town Press

McMahon, R., Malow, R. and Jennings, T. (2000) Personality, stress and social support in HIV risk prediction. *AIDS and Behavior* 4 (4): 399–410

MacPhail, C., Williams, B.C. and Campbell, C. (2002) Relative risk of HIV infection among young men and women in a South African township. *International Journal of STDs and AIDS* 13: 331–42

Mahlangu-Ngcobo, M. (2001) *AIDS in Africa: An African and Prophetic Perspective*. Baltimore, MD: Gateway Press

Makgoba, M. (1999) *African Renaissance*. Cape Town: Tafelberg Publishers.

Makgoba, M. (2000) HIV/AIDS: The perils of pseudoscience. *Science* 19 May, 288, 5469: 1171

Malik, R. (2000) Culture and emotions. In C. Squire (ed.) *Culture in Psychology*. London: Routledge

Mama. A. (2001) Talking about feminism in Africa (with Elaine Salo). *Agenda*, African Feminisms I, 50: 58–63

Mandela, N. (1995) *A Long Walk to Freedom*. London: Abacus

Mandela, N. (2000) Closing Address, 13th International AIDS Conference, Durban, 14 July. Online http://www.info.gov.za/speeches/2000/000714407p1001.htm. Accessed 10 October 2006

Mandela, W. (1985) *Part of my Soul went with him*. New York: Norton

Manganyi, C. (1989) *Treachery and Innocence*. Johannesburg: Ravan Press

Marshall, T. (1950) *Citizenship and Social Class and Other Essays*. Cambridge: Cambridge University Press

Mars-Jones, A. (1993) *Monopolies of Loss*. New York: Knopf

Matthews, C., Boon, H., Flisher, A. and Schaalma, H. (2006) Factors associated with teachers' implementation of AIDS education in Cape Town, South Africa. *AIDS Care* 18 (4): 388–92

Mattson, C., Bailey, R., Nnga, R., Poulussen, R. and Onyango, T. (2005) Acceptance of male circumcision and predictions of circumcision preference among women and men in Nyanza Province, Kenya. *AIDS Care* 17 (2): 182–94

Mays, V. and Cochran, S. (1988) Issues in the perception of AIDS risk and risk reduction activities by Black and Hispanic/Latina women. *American Psychologist* 43: 949–57

Mbali, M. (2003) HIV/AIDS policy-making in post-apartheid South Africa. In J. Daniel, A. Habib and R. Southall (eds) *State of the Nation: South Africa 2003–4*. Cape Town: HSRC Press.

Mbali, M. (2005) The Treatment Action Campaign and the History of Rights Based Patient-Driven HIV/Aids Activism in South Africa. *Centre for Civil Society* Research Report 29: 1–23

Mbeki, T. (1998) ANC has no financial stake in Virodene. March. Online http://www.anc.org.za/ancdocs/history/mbeki/1998/virodene.html. Accessed 10 October 2006

Mbeki, T. (2004a) When is good news bad news? *ANC Today* 4 (39), October: 1–7. Online http://www.anc.org.za/ancdocs/anctoday/2004/at39.htm. Accessed 20 August 2006

Mbeki , T. (2004b) Dislodging stereotypes. *ANC Today* 4 (42), October: 22–8. Online http://www.anc.org.za/ancdocs/anctoday/2004/at42.htm. Accessed 20 August 2006

Mbeki, T. (2005) Address of the President of South Africa, Thabo Mbeki, at the second joint sitting of the third democratic parliament, Cape Town, 11 February. Online http://www.info.gov.za/speeches/2005/05021110501001.htm. Accessed 20 August 2006

Mbembe, A. (2001) *On the Postcolony*. Berkeley, CA: University of California Press

Meares, R. (1996) South Africa AIDS musical has costly message. Reuters. Online http://www.aegis.com/news/re/1996/RE960376.html. Accessed 10 October 2006

Médecins sans Frontières (2003) Open Letter to the South African government, 12 February. Online http://www.accessmed-msf.org/prod/publications.asp?scntid=13220031455407&contenttype=PARA&. Accessed 20 August 2006

Médecins sans Frontières (2004) Antiretroviral therapy in primary health care: the experience of the Chiraduzulu programme in Malawi. MSF Malawi, July. Online http://www.accessmed-msf.org/documents/Chiradzulucasestudyjuly2004.pdf. Accessed 1 November 2006

Médecins sans Frontières (2005) *Effective Medical Care in Crisis Situations*. London: Médecins sans Frontières

Médecins sans Frontières and World Health Organisation (2003) *Antiretroviral therapy in primary health care: The experience from the Khayelitsha programme in South Africa*. World Health Organisation, Geneva

Mercer, K. (1994) *Welcome to the Jungle*. London: Routledge

Milford, C., Wassenaar, D. and Slack, C. (2006) Resources and needs of research ethics committees in Africa: Preparations for HIV vaccine trials. *IRB: Ethics and Human Research* 8 (2) March–April: 1–9. Online http://www.who.int/vaccine_research/diseases/hiv/docs/Resources_needs_HIV_vaccine_trials.pdf. Accessed 10 August 2006

Mishler, E. (1986) *Narrative Interviewing*. Cambridge, MA: Harvard University Press

Mkhise, N. (2004) Psychology: an African perspective. In D. Hook, N. Mkhise, P. Kiguwa and A. Collins (eds) *Critical Psychology*. Lansdowne, Western Cape: University of Cape Town Press

Moletsane, R., Morrell, R., Unterhalter, E., and Epstein, D. (2002) What kind of future can we make: Education, youth and HIV/AIDS. *Agenda* 53: 3–5

Monette, P. (1988) *Borrowed Time*. New York: Harper

Moodley, D. *et al.* (2000) The SAINT Trial: Nevirapine (NVP) versus Zidovudine (ZDV) + Lamivudine (3TC) in prevention of peripartum transmission. International AIDS conference, Durban, South Africa, July

Moore, G. and Beier, U. (eds) (1963) *Modern Poetry from Africa*. Harmondsworth: Penguin

Moore, O. (1996) *PWA: Looking AIDS in the Face*. London: Picador

Morojele, N., Brook, J. and Kachieng'A, M. (2006) Perceptions of social risk behaviours and substance abuse among adolescents in South Africa: A qualitative investigation. *AIDS Care* 18(3): 215–19

Morrell, R., Moletsane, R., Abdool Karim, Q., Epstein, D. and Unterhalter, E. (2002) The school setting: opportunities for integrating gender equality and HIV reduction interventions. *Agenda* 53: 11–21

Mostyn, B. (1985) The content analysis of qualitative data: a dynamic approach. In M. Brenner, J. Brown and D. Canter (eds) *The Research Interview: Uses and Approaches*. London: Academic Press

Motanyane, M. (1987) Two minutes. In A. Oosthuizen (ed.) *Sometimes When It Rains: Writings by South African Women*. London: Pandora

Mouffe, C. (1993) *The Return of the Political*. London: Verso

Mouffe, C. (1996) *Deconstruction and Pragmatism*. London: Routledge

Mphaphlele, E. (1959) *Down Second Avenue*. London: Faber & Faber

Mphaphlele, E. (1962) *The African Image*. London: Faber & Faber

Msimang, S. (2000) African renaissance: Where are the women? *Agenda* 41: 67–83

Mtathi, S. (2005) Queenstown Protest, 12 July – Summary of Events. Online www.tac.org.za/Documents/SummaryOfQueenstownEvents-20050803.doc. Accessed 20 August 2006

Mukamana, D. and Collins, A. (2006) Rape survivors of the Rwandan genocide. *International Journal of Critical Psychology* 16

Murphy, D., Steers, W. and Stritto, M. (2001) Maternal disclosure of mothers' HIV status to their young children. *Journal of Family Psychology* 15: 441–50

Murphy, T. and Poirier, S. (1993) *Writing AIDS*. New York: Columbia University Press

Naidoo, P. and Veriava, A. (2003) People before profits? A review of development and social change. *Development Update* 4 (4): 67–88

Naimak, T. (2006) Antiretroviral treatment in the Western Cape. CSSR Working Paper 161. August. Online http:///www.cssr.ac.za/index/htm. Accessed 20 August 2006.

National Institute of Health (2007) *NIH News*, 10.03. Online http://www.nih.gov/news/pr/mar2007/niaid-12.htm. Accessed 20 March 2007

Ndebele, N (1994) *Rediscovery of the Ordinary*. Johannesberg: COSAW

Ndebele, N. (2004) *The Cry of Winnie Mandela*. Banbury, Oxon: Ayebia Clarke Publishing

Ndingaye, X. (2005) An evaluation of the effects of poverty in Khayelitsha: A case study of Site C. MA thesis, Institute for Social Development, UWC. Online http://www.uwc.ac.za/library/theses/Ndingaye_x_z.pdf. Accessed 10 August 2006

Ndungane, N. (2005) Interview with Terri Gross. Fresh Air, National Public Radio, Philadelphia, 23 February. Online http://www.npr.org/templates/story/story.php?storyId=4509892. Accessed 10 August 2006

Nelson Mandela Foundation/HSRC (2002). *South African National HIV Prevalence, Behavioural Risks and Mass Media*. Cape Town: HSRC Press

Nkosi, L. (1959) Why 'Bloke' baled out. *Contact* 11 July. Online http://disa.nu.ac.za/Content/Ct/Ctv2n1459/Ctv2n1459.pdf. Accessed 1 April 2007

Nuwagaba-Biribonwoha, H., Mayon-White, R., Okong, P., Carpenter, L. and Jenkinson (2006) Impact on HIV on maternal quality of life in Uganda. *AIDS Care* 18(6): 614–20

Odets, W. (1995) *In the Shadow of the Epidemic*. London: Cassell

Office of the Public Protector (1996) *Report No 1 (Special Report) Investigation of the Play Sarafina II*. June. Online http://www.polity.org.za/html/govt/pubprot/report1a.html?rebookmark=1. Accessed 10 August 2006

Ogbonnaya, N. (1994) Person as community: an African understanding of the person as an intrapsychic community. *Journal of Black Psychology* 20: 75–87

Ogundipe-Leslie, M. (1994) *Recreating Ourselves: African Women and Critical Transformation*. Lawrenceville, NJ: Africa World Press

Oloka-Onyango, J. and Tamale, S. (1995) The personal is political, or why women's rights are indeed human rights: an African perspective on international feminism. *Human Rights Quarterly* 17 (4): 691–731

Onyango, M., and Majola, M. (2006) Living with HIV: Men's role in care, support, testing, treatment and gender equity. International AIDS Conference, July, Toronto

Olley, B., Zeier, M., Seedat, S. and Stein, D. (2005) Post-traumatic stress disorder among recently diagnosed patients with HIV/AIDS in South Africa. *AIDS Care* 17 (5): 550–7

Oosthuisen, M. and Hexham, I. (1989) *Afro-christian Religion and Healing in Southern Africa*. Lewiston, NY: E. Mellen Press

Oppenheimer, J. and Reckit, H. (1997) *Acting on AIDS*. London: Serpent's Tail

Orrell, C., Bangsber, D., Badri, M. and Wood, R. (2003) Adherence is not a barrier to successful antiretroviral therapy in South Africa. *AIDS* 17: 1367–75

O'Sullivan, S. (2000) Uniting across boundaries: HIV positive women in global perspective. *Agenda* 44: 25–31

Outwater, A., Abrahams, N. and Campbell, J. (2005) Intentional violence and HIV/AIDS: Intersections and prevention. *Journal of Black Studies* 53 (4): 135–54

Ouzgane, L. and Morrell, R. (2005) *African Masculinities*. London: Palgrave Macmillan

Overseas Development Institute (2006) *Scaling up on HIV/AIDS*. Online http://www.odi.org.uk/speeches/aids_06/7%20June/index.html. Accessed 20 August 2006

Papa, M., Singhal, A., Law, S., Pant, S., Sood, S., Rogers, E. and Shefner-Rogers, C.L. (2001) Entertainment-education and social change: An analysis of parasocial interaction, social learning, collective efficacy, and paradoxical communication. *Journal of Communication* 50 (4): 31–55

Parker, I. (1998) *Social Construction, Discourse and Realism*. London: Sage

Pato, L. (1997) Indigenisation and liberation. A challenge to theology in the southern African context. *Journal of Theology for Southern Africa* 99: 40–6. Online http://web.uct.ac.za/depts/ricsa/j99pato.htm. Accessed 20 September 2006

Patton, C. (1991) *Inventing AIDS*. London: Routledge

Patton, C. (1993) 'With champagne and roses': Women at risk from/in AIDS discourse. In C. Squire (ed.) *Women and AIDS*. London: Sage

Patton, C. (1994) *Last Served? Gendering the Pandemic*. New York: Taylor & Francis.

Patton, C. (2002) *Globalising AIDS*. Minneapolis, MN: Minnesota University Press

Peires, J. (1989) *The Dead Will Arise: Nongqawuse and the Great Xhosa Cattle-Killing Movement of 1865–7*. Bloomington, IN: Indiana University Press

Peltzer, K. Mngqundaniso, N. and Petros, G. (2006) HIV/AIDS/STI/TB knowledge, beliefs and practices of traditional healers in KwaZulu-Natal, South Africa. *AIDS Care* 18 (6): 608–13

Phillips, H. (2001) AIDS in the context of South Africa's epidemic history. *South African Historical Journal* 45: 11–26

Piot, P. (2001) Address to the World Conferences against Racism, Durban. Online http://www.unhchr.ch/huricane/huricane.nsf/(Symbol)/OHCHR.WCAR.PR.22.En?OpenDocument. Accessed 1 November 2006

Plummer, K. (1995) *Telling Sexual Stories*. London: Sage

Plummer, K. (2001) *Documents of Life 2*. London: Sage

Plummer, K. (2003) *Intimate Citizenship*. London: Sage

Poku, N. and Whiteside, A. (2004) *The Political Economy of AIDS in Africa*. London: Ashgate

Policy Coordination and Advisory Services (2006) A Nation in the Making Social Sector, The Presidency. Online http://www.info.gov.za/otherdocs/2006/socioreport.pdf#search=%22a%20nation%20in%20the%20making%22. Accessed 20 August 2006

Population Action International (2006) Why condoms are under seige. (Transcript). Online http://www.populationaction.org/news/Teleconf_Transcript1.pdf. Accessed 10 August 2006

Preston, R. (1994) *The Hot Zone*. New York: Random House

Pretorius, H. and Jafta, L. (1997) A branch springs out: African Initiated Churches. In R. Elphick and R. Davenport (eds) *Christianity in South Africa*. Berkeley, CA: University of California Press, 212–16

Putnam, R. (2000) *Bowling Alone: The Collapse and Revivial of American Community*. New York: Simon & Schuster

Ratele, K. (2004) About black psychology. In D. Hook, N. Mkhise, P. Kiguwa and A. Collins (eds) *Critical Psychology*. Lansdowne, Western Cape: University of Cape Town Press

Ratele, K. and Shefer, T. (2002) Stigma in the social construction of sexually transmitted diseases. In D. Hook and G. Eagle (eds) *Psychopathology and Social Prejudice*. Cape Town: University of Cape Town Press

Reeler, A. (1998) Epidemic violence and the community: A Zimbabwean case study. *Journal of Social Development in Africa* 13: 41–51

Reparation and Rehabilitation Committee (2003) *Report of the Reparation and Rehabilitation Committee. Implications and concluding comments*. Online http://www.info.gov.za/otherdocs/2003/trc/2_7.pdf. Accessed 1 November 2006

Reproductive Health Research Unit/loveLife (2004) *HIV and Sexual Behaviour among young South Africans: A National Survey of 15–24 year olds*. University of the

Witwatersrund. Online http://www.kff.org/southafrica/upload/HIV-and-Sexual-Behaviour-Among-Young-South-Africans-A-National-Survey-of-15–24-Year-Olds.pdf. Accessed 10 August 2006

Richardson, D. (1987) *Women and the AIDS Crisis*. New York: Methuen

Ricoeur, P. (1984) *Time and Narrative*. Chicago: University of Chicago Press

Rieder, I. and Ruppelt, P. (1989) *Matters of Life and Death: Women Speak about AIDS*. London: Time Warner

Riessman, C. (1993) *Narrative Analysis*. New York: Sage

Robins, S. (2004) 'Long live Zackie, long live!' AIDS activism, science and citizenship after apartheid. *Journal of Southern African Studies* 30 (3): 651–72

Rose, N. and Novas, C. 2004. Biological citizenship. In A. Ong, S. Collier and S. Blackwell (eds) *Global Assemblages: Technology, Politics, and Ethics as Anthropological Problems*. Oxford: Blackwell

Rosen, S. Vincent, J., MacLeod, W., Fox, M., Thea, D. and Simon, J. (2004) The cost of HIV/AIDS to businesses in southern Africa. *AIDS* 18: 317–24

Rounaq, J. (1995) *The Elusive Agenda: Mainstreaming Women*. London: Zed Books

Russell, D. (1989) *Lives of Courage*. New York: Basic Books

Sanneh, L. (1983) *West African Christianity: The Religious Impact*. Maryknoll, NY: Orbis Books

Sarason, L., Sarason, B. and Pierce, G. (1990) Social support: The search for theory. *Journal of Social and Clinical Psychology* 9: 133–142

Scheepers, I., Christofides, N., Goldstein, S., Usdin, S., Patel, D. and Japhet, G. (2004) Evaluating health communication – a holistic overview of the impact of Soul City IV. *Health Promotion Journal of Australia* 15 (2): 121–9

Schmidt, C. and Goggin, K. (2006) Disclosure, social support and depression: The pattern among HIV+ women. Forthcoming. Online http://www.ISCPubs.com/articles/ad/c0203sch.pdf. Accessed 1 April 2007

Searle, J. (1969) *Speech Acts*. Cambridge: Cambridge University Press

Selikow, T., Zulu, B. and Cedras, E. (2002) The ingagara, the regte and the cherry: HIV/AIDS and youth culture in contemporary urban townships. *Agenda*. 53: 22–32

Shaikh, N., Abdullah, F., Lombard, C., Smit, L., Bradshaw, D. and Makubalo, L. (2006) Masking through averages – intraprovincial heterogeneity in HIV prevalence within the Western Cape. *South African Medical Journal* 96 (6): 538–43

Shea, D. (1968) *Spiritual Autobiography in Early America*. Princeton, NJ: Princeton University Press

Shilts, Randy (1988) *And the Band Played on*. New York: St Martin's Press

Shisana, O., Rehle, T., Simbayi, L., Parker, W., Zuma, K., Bhana, A., Connolly, C., Jooste, S. and Pillay, V. (2005) *South African National HIV Prevalence, HIV Incidence, Behaviour and Communication Survey*. Cape Town: HSRC Press

Shweder, R. (1991) *Thinking Through Cultures*. Cambridge, MA: Harvard University Press

Sigogo, T. and Tso Modipa, O. (2004) Critical reflections on community and psychology in South Africa. In D. Hook, N. Mkhise, P. Kiguwa and A. Collins (eds) *Critical Psychology*. Lansdowne, Western Cape: University of Cape Town Press

Singhal A., Usdin, S., Scheepers, E., Goldstein, S. and Japhet, G. (2004) Harnessing the education-entertainment strategy in Africa: The Soul City intervention in South Africa. In C. Okigbo and F. Eribo (eds) *Development and Communication in Africa*. Lanham, MD: Rowman and Littlefield

Skocpol, T. (1994) *Social Revolutions in the Modern World*. New York: Cambridge University Press

Skjelsbaek, I. (2006) Narrated social identities of women who experienced rape in Bosnia-Herzegovina. *Feminism and Psychology* 16 (4): 373–404

Skogmar, S., Shkaeley, D., Lam, M., Daniell, J., Andersson, R., Tshandu, N., Odón, A., Roberts, S. and Venter, F. (2006) Effects of antiretroviral treatment and counselling on disclosure of HIV serostatus in Johannesburg, South Africa. *AIDS Care* 18 (7): 725–30

Skordis, J. and Nattrass, Nicoli (2002 Paying to waste lives: The affordability of reducing mother-to-child transmission of HIV in South Africa. *Journal of Health Economics* 21 (3): 405–21

Solidarity Peace Trust (2004) *An Account of the Exodus of a Nation's People.* Port Shepstone, KwaZulu-Natal. Online http://209.85.129.104/search?q=cache:cx5i8yx Y1uMJ:www.solidaritypeacetrust.org/reports/no_war.pdf+sawima+3+million+sun day+times&hl=en&gl=uk&ct=clnk&cd=10. Accessed 10 October 2006

Song, Y. and Ingram, K. (2002) Unsupportive social interactions, availability of social support, and coping: Their relationship to mood disturbance among African Americans living with HIV. *Journal of Social and Personal Relationships* 19 (1): 67–85

Sontag, S. (2001) *Illness as Metaphor and AIDS and its Metaphors.* New York: Picador

Soul City/MarkData (2005) Evaluation, Soul City Series 6. Parktown Soul City Institute. Online http://www.soulcity.org.za/downloads/Series%206%20Evaluation. pdf. Accessed 10 August 2006

South African Broadcasting Corporation (2006) *Special Assignment: A Better Life?* 6 March. Transcript. Online http:// www.sabcnews.com/specialassignment/better script.html. Accessed 10 October 2006

South African Commission for Gender Equality and the South African Human Rights Commission (2001). Report on Consultative Conference on Virginity Testing held in South Africa on 12 June 2000

Spacks, P. (1985) *Gossip.* New York: Knopf

Spivak, G. (1990)*The Postcolonial Critic: Interviews, Strategies, Dialogues.* London: Routledge

Spivak, G. (1994 [1985]) Can the Subaltern Speak? In P. Williams and L. Chrisman (eds) *Colonial Discourse and Postcolonial Theory: A Reader.* Hemel Hempstead: Harvester Wheatsheaf

Squire, C. (1993) *Women and AIDS: Psychological Perspectives.* London: Sage

Squire, C. (1997) AIDS Panic. In Jane Ussher (ed.) *Body Talk.* London: Routledge

Squire, C. (1999) 'Neighbors who might become friends': Selves, genres and citizenship in stories of HIV. *The Sociological Quarterly* 40 (1): 109–37

Squire, C. (2003) Can an HIV positive woman find true love? Romance in the stories of women living with HIV. *Feminism and Psychology* 3 (1): 73–100

Squire, C. (2004) 'I am still your sister': Psychology, women and HIV. *Psychology of Women Review* 6

Squire, C. (2005) Reading Narratives. *Group Analysis* 38 (1): 91–107

Squire, C. (2006) Feeling entitled: HIV, entitlement feelings and citizenship. In P. 6., S. Radstone, C. Squire and A. Treacher (eds) *Public Emotions.* London: Palgrave Macmillan

Squire, C. (forthcoming) From experience – centred to culturally-oriented narratives. In M. Andrews, C. Squire and M. Tamboukou (eds) *Doing Narrative Research.* London: Sage

Staiano, K. (1992) *The Semiotic Perspective.* In J. Lachmund and G. Stollberg (eds) *The Social Construction of Illness.* Stuttgart: Franz Steiner Verlag

Statistics South Africa (2001) Census 2001. Online http://www.statssa.gov.za/census 01/html/default.asp. Accessed 31 July 2006

Statistics South Africa (2005) Labour force survey, September 2005. Online http://www.statssa.gov.za/PublicationsHTML/P0210September2005/html/P0210Se ptember2005.html. Accessed 31 July 2006

Stenson, A., Charalambou, S., Dwadwa, T., Pemba, L., Du Toit, J., Baggelery, R., Grant, A. and Churchyard, G. (2005) Evaluation of antiretroviral therapy (ART)-related counselling in a workplace-based ART implementation programme, South Africa. *AIDS Care* 17 (8): 949–57

Stromberg, P. (1993) *Language and Self-Transformation*. Cambridge: Cambridge University Press

Tambo, O. (1987) *Oliver Tambo Speaks*. London: Heinemann

Tarakeshwar, N., Khan, N. and Sikkema, K. (2006) A relationship-based framework of spirituality for individuals with HIV. *AIDS and Behavior* 10 (1): 59–70

Tarrow, S. (2005) *The New Transnational Activism*. Cambridge: Cambridge University Press

Todorov, T. (1990) *Genres in Discourse*. Cambridge: Cambridge University Press

Toscano O. (2002) *Colors: The Benetton Campaigns*. London: Scriptum Editions

Treatment Action Campaign (2004) Commemoration rally for Lorna Mlofana in Khayelitsha Newsletter 14 December. Online http://www.tac.org.za/newsletter/ 2004/ns15_12_2004b.html. Accessed 10 October 2006

Treatment Action Campaign (2005) Matthias Rath and TAC's efforts to stop his harmful activities. Online http://www.tac.org.za/rath.html. Accessed 10 October 2006

Treatment Action Campaign (2006) Statement on the death of Nozipho Bhengu 24 May. Online http://www.tac.org.za/nl20060524a.html. Accessed 10 October 2006

Treichler, P. (1988) AIDS, homophobia and biomedical discourse: An epidemic of signification. In D. Crimp (ed.) *AIDS: Cultural Analysis/Cultural Activism* Boston, MA: MIT Press

Treichler, P. (1999) *How to Have Theory in an Epidemic: Cultural Chronicles of AIDS*. Durham, NC: Duke University Press

Trinatapoli, J. and Regnerus, M. (2005) Risk behaviours among men: initial results from a panel study in rural sub-Saharan Africa. PCR Working Paper Series. Online http://www.prc.utexas.edu/working_papers/wp_pdf/04-05-05.pdf. Accessed 20 March 2007

Troiden, R. (1979). Becoming homosexual: a model of gay identity acquisition. *Psychiatry* 42: 362–73

Truth and Reconciliation Commission and Tutu, D. (1999) *Truth and Reconciliation Commission of South Africa Report*. London: Palgrave Macmillan

Tutu, D. (2006) [1989] *The Words of Desmond Tutu*. New York: Newmarket Press

UNAIDS (2004) Report on the global AIDS epidemic. Online http://www.unaids. org/bangkok2004/GAR2004_00_en.htm. Accessed 20 March 2007

UNAIDS (2005) *AIDS in Africa: Three Scenarios to 2025*. Online http://www.unaids. org/unaids_resources/images/AIDSScenarios/AIDS-scenarios-2025_section1_ en.pdf. Accessed 31 July 2006

UNAIDS (2006) Report on the global AIDS epidemic. Online http://www.unaids. org/en/HIV_data/2006GlobalReport/default.asp. Accessed 31 July 2006

UNAIDS/WHO (2006) AIDS Epidemic Update. Online http://www.unaids.org/en/ HIV_data/epi2006/default.asp

UNICEF/World Health Organisation (2006) *Immunisation Summary*. New York: United Nations Publications. Online http://www.unicef.org/publications/files/Immunization_Summary_2006.pdf. Accessed 10 October 2006

United Nations (1997) *Gender Mainstreaming*. Online http://www.un.org/women watch/daw/csw/GMS.PDF. Accessed 20 October 2006

United Nations (2006) *World Report on Violence Against Children*. Geneva. Online http://www.unviolencestudy.org/. Accessed 20 October 2006

Uys, P. (2003) *Elections and Erections: A Memoir of Fear and Fun*. South Africa: Zebra Press

Vanlandingham, M., Im-Em, W. and Yokota, F. (2006) Access to treatment and care associated with HIV infection among members of AIDS support groups in Thailand. *AIDS Care* 18 (7): 637–46

Van Vlaenderen, H. and Neves, D. (2004) Participatory Action Research and local knowledge in community contexts. In D. Hook, N. Mkhise, P. Kiguwa and A. Collins (eds) *Critical Psychology*. Lansdowne, Western Cape: University of Cape Town Press

Walch, S., Roetzer, L. and Minnett, T. (2006) Support group participation among persons with HIV: demographic characteristics and perceived barriers. *AIDS Care* 18 (4): 284–9

Wallerstein, I. (2004) *World Systems Analysis: An Introduction*. Durham, NC: Duke University Press

Walzer, M. (1983) *Spheres of Justice*. New York: Basic Books.

Watney, S. (1990) Missionary positions: AIDS, Africa and race. In R. Ferguson, M. Gever, T. Minh-Ha and C. West (eds) *Out There*. Cambridge, MA: MIT Press

Watney, S. (1991) Representing AIDS. In T. Boffin and S. Gupta (eds) *Ecstatic Antibodies*. London: River's Oram

Watney, S. (1994) *Practices of Freedom*. London: Rivers Oram

Watney, S. (2000) *Imagine Hope*. London: Routledge

Webb, B. (2006) AIDS orphanages rethink. *Daily News*, 28 July: 3

Weeks, J. (1985) *Sexuality and its Discontents*. London: Routledge & Kegan Paul

Weeks, J. (1995) *Invented Moralities: Sexual Values in the Age of Uncertainty*. London: Polity Press

West, C. (1989) *The American Evasion of Philosophy*. Madison, WI: University of Wisconsin Press

White, E. (2000) *The Married Man*. New York: Knopf.

Whiteside, A. and Sunter, C. (2000) *AIDS: The Challenge for South Africa*. Johannesburg: Human and Rousseau

Wilbraham, L. (2004) Discursive practice: Analysing a *lovelines* text on sex communication for parents. In D. Hook, N. Mkhise, P. Kiguwa and A. Collins (eds) *Critical Psychology*. Lansdowne, Western Cape: University of Cape Town Press

Wilkinson, R. (2005) *The Impact of Inequality*. London: Routledge

Williams, B., Lloyd-Smith, J., Gouws, E., Hankins, C., Getz, W., Hargrove, J., deZoysa, I., Dye, C. and Auvert, B. (2006) The potential impact of male circumcision on HIV in sub-Saharan Africa. PloS Medicine 3 (7). Online http://medicine. plosjournals.org/perlserv/?request=get-document&doi=10.1371/journal.pmed. 0030262. Accessed 1 April 2007

Williams, B., Lloyd-Smith, J. Gouws, E., Hankin, C., Getz, W., Hargrove, J., deZoysa, I., Dye, C. and Auvert, B. Gouws, E., Colvin, M., Sitas, F., Ramjee, G. and Karim, S. (2000) Patterns of infection: using age prevalence data to understand the epidemic of HIV in South Africa. *South African Journal of Science* 96, June: 1–9

Williamson, J. (1989) Every virus tells a story. In E. Carter and S. Watney (eds) *Taking Liberties*. London: Serpent's Tail

Wojnarowicz, D. (1991) *Close to the Knives*. New York: Vintage

Wolfe, W., Weiser, S., Leiter, K., Steward, W., Korte, P., Phaladze, N., Iacopino, V., Heiser, M. *et al*. (2006) Impact of universal access to antiretroviral therapy on HIV stigma in Botswana. International AIDS Conference, Toronto, July.

Woods. T., Antoni, M., Ironson, G. and Kling, D. (1999) Religiosity is associated with affective status in symptomatic HIV-infected African-American women. *Journal of Health Psychology* 4 (3): 317–26

World Health Organisation (2003) *Traditional Medicine: Report by the Secretariat*. Geneva: World Health Organisation. Online http://www.who.int/gb/ebwha/pdf_ files/WHA56/ea5618.pdf#search=%22self-care%20world%20health%20organisation %22. Accessed 30 August 2006

World Health Organisation (2004) Position statement on the safety and quality of oral polio vaccine (opv) supplied to Nigeria. Geneva: World Health Organisation. Online http://www.who.int/countries/nga/areas/polio/opv_position_210104.pdf. Accessed 31 July 2006

World Health Organisation (2005) Interim WHO Clinical Staging of HIV/AIDS and HIV/AIDS Case Definitions for Surveillance, African Region. Geneva: World Health Organisation. Online http://www.who.int/hiv/pub/guidelines/clinicalstaging. pdf. Accessed 31 July 2006

World Health Organisation (2006a) Progress on Access to HIV Antiretroviral Therapy: A report on '3 by 5' and beyond. Geneva: World Health Organisation. Online http:// www.who.int/hiv/progreport2006_en.pdf. Accessed 31 July 2006

World Health Organisation (2006b) WHO HIV and Infant Feeding Technical Consultation. Held on behalf of the Inter-agency Task Team (IATT) on Prevention of HIV Infections in Pregnant Women, Mothers and their Infants. Geneva, 25–7 October 2006: Consensus Statement. Geneva: World Health Organisation: World Health Organisation. Online http://www.who.int/child-adolescent-health/New_ Publications/NUTRITION/consensus-statement.pdf. Accessed 10 April 2007

World Health Organisation (2007) Towards Universal Access: Scaling up priority HIV/AIDs interventions in the health sector: progress report, April 2007. Geneva: World Health Organisation. Online http://www.who.int/hiv/mediacentre/universal_ accesss_progress__report_en.pdf. Accessed 1 June 2007.

Young, I. (1990) *Justice and the Politics of Difference*. Princeton, NJ: Princeton University Press

Index

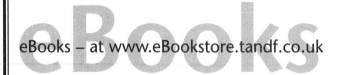

eBooks – at www.eBookstore.tandf.co.uk

A library at your fingertips!

eBooks are electronic versions of printed books. You can store them on your PC/laptop or browse them online.

They have advantages for anyone needing rapid access to a wide variety of published, copyright information.

eBooks can help your research by enabling you to bookmark chapters, annotate text and use instant searches to find specific words or phrases. Several eBook files would fit on even a small laptop or PDA.

NEW: Save money by eSubscribing: cheap, online access to any eBook for as long as you need it.

Annual subscription packages

We now offer special low-cost bulk subscriptions to packages of eBooks in certain subject areas. These are available to libraries or to individuals.

For more information please contact webmaster.ebooks@tandf.co.uk

We're continually developing the eBook concept, so keep up to date by visiting the website.

www.eBookstore.tandf.co.uk

Related titles from Routledge

Culture, Society and Sexuality: A Reader

Edited by Richard Parker and Peter Aggleton

This new and revised edition brings together and makes accessible a broad and international selection of readings to provide insights into the social, cultural, political and economic dimensions of sexuality and relationships, and emerging discourses around sexual and reproductive rights.

Clearly structured and presented, the book makes an extremely useful reference for students and researchers. Section one focuses on the social and cultural construction of sexuality as an emerging field of inquiry, and examines some of the most important theoretical insights and areas of investigation that have emerged. Section two links research on the construction of sexuality to a growing body of work on gender and sexuality in relation to a wide range of practical issues and contemporary social policy debates.

It is an essential reader for students, researchers, activists, health workers and service providers, who daily confront practical and policy issues related to sexuality, sexual health and sexual rights.

Hb: 978–0–415–40455–6
Pb: 978–0–415–40456–3

Available at all good bookshops
For ordering and further information please visit:
www.routledge.com

Related titles from Routledge

21st Century Sexualities:
Contemporary issues in health, education, and rights

Edited by Gilbert Herdt and Cymene Howe

Exploring sexuality in the twenty-first century, this unique book collects together more than fifty timely and accessible contributions to create a wide-ranging and compelling picture of contemporary American sexuality.

Incorporating the latest cutting-edge controversies, theory and methodological material from the major domains of sexual education, sexual health, sexual rights, and globalization, this book includes a superb editorial overview that opens up the field for students and teachers alike.

This anthology will be an invaluable supplement to all levels of students and researchers interested in sexuality across a range of disciplines, including anthropology, sociology, gender and sexuality studies and politics.

Hb: 978–0–415–77306–5
Pb: 978–0–415–77307–2

Available at all good bookshops
For ordering and further information please visit:
www.routledge.com

Printed and bound by CPI Group (UK) Ltd, Croydon, CR0 4YY

01/11/2024

01782631-0002